The ASQ User's Guide

Second Edition

ASQ™

The ASQ User's Guide
Second Edition

ASQ™

by

Jane Squires, Ph.D.

LaWanda Potter, M.S.

and

Diane Bricker, Ph.D.

Early Intervention Program
Center on Human Development
University of Oregon, Eugene

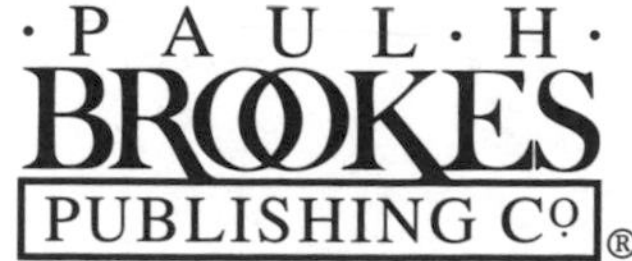

Baltimore • London • Sydney

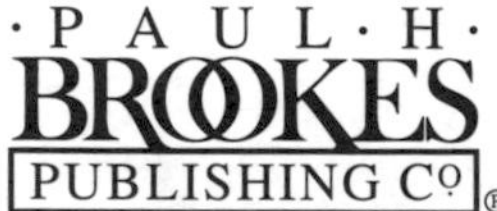

Paul H. Brookes Publishing Co.
Post Office Box 10624
Baltimore, Maryland 21285-0624

www.brookespublishing.com

See the end of this guide for information about accompanying products in the ASQ system.

Typeset by Barton Matheson Willse & Worthington, Baltimore, Maryland.
Manufactured in the United States of America by Versa Press, East Peoria, Illinois.

Second printing, December 1999.
Third printing, August 2001. This printing was updated to include references to the ASQ:SE © 2001.
Fourth printing, July 2002.
Fifth printing, May 2004. This printing was updated to include references to *ASQ CD-ROM* and *Edades y Etapas CD-ROM* (© 1999) and the videotapes *ASQ Scoring & Referral* and *ASQ:SE in Practice* (© 2004).
Sixth printing, September 2005. This printing has been updated to include additional suggested readings (pp. 109–110) and to list revised cutoff scores for nine intervals.
Seventh printing, October 2006.

Library of Congress Cataloging-in-Publication Data

Squires, Jane.
The ASQ user's guide / by Jane Squires, LaWanda Potter, and Diane Bricker.—2nd ed.
p. cm.
Originally published: Baltimore, MD : Paul H. Brookes, 1995.
Includes bibliographical references and index.
ISBN-13: 978-1-55766-367-2
ISBN-10: 1-55766-367-X
1. Child Development—Testing. 2. Infants—Development—Testing. 3. Child development deviations—Diagnosis. I. Potter, LaWanda. II. Bricker, Diane D. III. Title.
RJ51.D48B75 1999 Suppl.
618.92'0075—dc21 98-43539

British Library Cataloguing in Publication data are available from the British Library.

CONTENTS

ASQ™

List of Tables and Figures

APPENDIX F

About the Authors

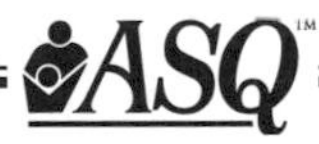

The ASQ system, including the *Ages & Stages Questionnaires* (English, Spanish, and French versions); *The ASQ User's Guide,* the *Ages & Stages Questionnaires: Social-Emotional* (English and Spanish versions); *The ASQ:SE User's Guide; ASQ CD-ROM* and *ASQ:SE CD-ROM* (English and Spanish versions); and the videotapes *ASQ Scoring & Referral, The Ages & Stages Questionnaires on a Home Visit,* and *ASQ:SE in Practice,* were developed by the following authors:

Diane Bricker, Ph.D., Professor Emerita and Former Director, Early Intervention Program, Center on Human Development, University of Oregon, Eugene, Oregon

Dr. Bricker is former director of the Early Intervention Program at the Center on Human Development, University of Oregon. She is Professor Emerita of special education, focusing on the fields of early intervention and communication. Dr. Bricker has been the primary author of the *Ages & Stages Questionnaires* and directed research activities on the ASQ system since 1980. Dr. Bricker has published extensively on assessment/evaluation and personnel preparation in early intervention.

Jane Squires, Ph.D., Professor and Director, Early Intervention Program, Center on Human Development, University of Oregon, Eugene, Oregon

Dr. Squires is a professor in special education, focusing on the field of early intervention, at the University of Oregon. Dr. Squires has directed several research studies on the *Ages & Stages Questionnaires* and has also directed national outreach training activities related to developmental screening and the involvement of parents in the monitoring of their child's development. In addition to her interests in screening and tracking, Dr. Squires directs a master's-level rural personnel preparation program, teaches classes in the early intervention area, and is Associate Director of the Center for Excellence in Developmental Disabilities.

Linda Mounts, M.A., Child Development Specialist, Regional Center of the East Bay, Oakland, California

Ms. Mounts is an infant development specialist and has worked for many years in clinical and research settings with infants and toddlers. While at the Center on Human Development, University of Oregon, she assisted with development and research on the *Ages & Stages Questionnaires.* She is employed by the Regional Center of the East Bay in northern California, evaluating young children from birth to 3 years of age.

LaWanda Potter, M.S., Research Assistant, Early Intervention Program, Center on Human Development, University of Oregon, Eugene, Oregon

Ms. Potter is a research assistant at the Early Intervention Program, Center on Human Development, University of Oregon. She has been involved with several research studies on the *Ages & Stages Questionnaires,* including questionnaire revisions, data analysis, and documentation. She has also provided outreach training on the *Ages & Stages Questionnaires* system across the United States. Ms. Potter is the co-developer of the videotape *The Ages & Stages Questionnaires on a Home Visit.*

Robert Nickel, M.D., Associate Professor of Pediatrics, Department of Pediatrics, and Medical Director, Child Development and Rehabilitation Center, Oregon Health Sciences University, Eugene, Oregon

Dr. Nickel is an associate professor of pediatrics in the Department of Pediatrics and at the Child Development and Rehabilitation Center (CDRC), Oregon Health Sciences University, and he is the medical director of the Eugene office at CDRC. He has been instrumental in the production of other materials related to developmental monitoring activities, including the *Infant Motor Screen* (screen test/manual and videotape) and *Developmental Screening for Infants 0–3 Years of Age* (manual and videotape), part of a training program for primary health care professionals. As a developmental pediatrician, he attends a number of clinics for children with special health care needs in the Portland and Eugene CDRC offices and at outreach sites.

Elizabeth Twombly, M.S., Research Assistant, Early Intervention Program, Center on Human Development, University of Oregon, Eugene, Oregon

Ms. Twombly is a research assistant at the Early Intervention Program, Center on Human Development, University of Oregon. She provides training and technical assistance to state agencies on the ASQ system. She has been involved in several research studies on the ASQ, including the development of additional intervals for the second edition.

Jane Farrell, M.S., Early Childhood Special Educator, Air Force Services for Exceptional Children, Wiesbaden, Germany

Ms. Farrell was the project coordinator of the ASQ Outreach Project, a federally funded outreach grant providing training and technical assistance on the use of the ASQ for interagency early childhood screening, monitoring, and tracking efforts. She works in Germany at an Air Force clinic providing early intervention services to children from birth to 3 years of age and their families. Ms. Farrell is the co-developer of the videotape *The Ages & Stages Questionnaires on a Home Visit.*

PREFACE

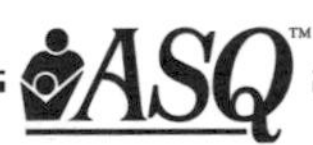

As the fields of early intervention and early childhood special education moved into the 1980s, a number of important changes were on the horizon. In particular, we, like many others, saw three significant and interrelated needs. First, there was a great need for parents and family members to become genuinely involved in the assessment, intervention, and evaluation activities surrounding their infants and young children who were at risk or had disabilities. Second, there was a clearly articulated need for tests or procedures that would monitor the development of infants who were thought to be at high risk for developing problems as a result of medical, biological, or environmental factors, or a combination of these factors. Third, there was growing pressure, spurred by diminishing resources, to find effective yet economical means to serve growing numbers of children who were at risk or had disabilities and their families. Our awareness of these problems set the stage for the development of the *Ages & Stages Questionnaires* (ASQ).[1]

The impetus for the development of the ASQ system came from several sources. The first source was the belief of many, if not most, scientists, practitioners, and parents that early detection of developmental problems is essential to timely and effective intervention. Second was the consistent finding that biological or medical indicators (e.g., prematurity, low birth weight, small-for-gestational-age) are not reliable predictors of subsequent infant outcomes (Parmelee & Cohen, 1985). An infant who is premature and has health problems during the neonatal period will not necessarily have developmental problems at age 3, 4, or older. Major longitudinal studies of infants considered at risk for developmental delay consistently report that socioeconomic, rather than biological, factors are the best indicators of future problems (Blackman, 1996; Sameroff, 1981; Werner & Smith, 1992).

A third impetus for the development of the ASQ system was the prevalent use of a multidisciplinary team evaluation model for monitoring the development of designated populations of children. This model requires that children be brought to an evaluation center for a multidisciplinary examination conducted by a group of highly trained professionals. Using this model, infants tend to be seen only once or at widely spaced intervals (e.g., yearly). Given the dynamic nature of development, systems that evaluate an infant at only one point in time or at extended time intervals seem likely to be ineffec-

[1]Previously called the Infant/Child Monitoring Questionnaires.

tive in the timely identification of children who may require intervention services. Problems can arise in children at any point in their developmental trajectory, requiring that effective monitoring systems assess children at reasonable time intervals.

In addition, multidisciplinary team evaluations tend to rely primarily on professional judgment and tend to seek little information about the child's behavior from parents or family members. Parents were seen as the recipients of information and were expected to contribute little to the understanding of their child, except for a recitation of past health and general family experiences. In addition to infrequent evaluations and exclusion of parents' input about their child, the use of highly skilled professional teams to monitor the development of large groups of infants at risk for developmental delay is expensive. The expense is particularly troublesome given that much of the team's time is likely to be spent evaluating children whose development is progressing without problem. It has been consistently reported that approximately 30% of the infants identified with a biological or medical risk factor (e.g., prematurity) require some form of intervention (Widerstom & Nickel, 1997). Although it seems useful to monitor the development of risk populations, it seems inappropriate to use expensive, highly skilled professionals to do so.

We believe that the development of all infants and young children should be consistently monitored; however, that elusive goal remains a challenge (Bricker, 1996). Until the challenge is met, the development of infants and young children experiencing biological, medical, or environmental risk factors should be periodically evaluated; however, the problems described above strongly suggested to us the need for change. Thus, in 1979, we began work on a monitoring system designed to circumvent, or at least attenuate, the difficulties of prediction, timeliness, accuracy, and cost. Our goal was to develop a system that was both effective and affordable. Specifically, the evaluations should occur at well-spaced intervals, the procedure should accurately identify children in need of further evaluation, the system should be easy to set up and maintain, the systematic inclusion of information from parents or caregivers should occur, and the monitoring should be economical.

The criteria indicated above set the parameters for the type of system we were interested in developing. Inspiration for the *Ages & Stages Questionnaires* came from an article published in 1979 by Hilda Knobloch and her colleagues (Knobloch, Stevens, Malone, Ellison, & Risemburg, 1979). In this study, a 36-item questionnaire with items derived from the Revised Gesell Developmental Examination (Knobloch, Stevens, & Malone, 1980) representing the developmental period from 20 to 32 weeks was mailed to the parents of more than 526 28-week-old infants considered at high risk for developmental problems. The questionnaires were completed, returned, and scored to classify the infants as normal, abnormal, or questionable. At 40 weeks, the infants were brought to a clinic for a professional evaluation. Knobloch et al. (1979) reported that according to the professional evaluation, parents and professionals were in general agreement about the classification of the infants. The success of this study led us to reason that it might be possible to develop a dynamic monitoring system for infants and children that relied essentially on feedback from parents or primary caregivers.

By the end of 1979, a set of six questionnaires was developed to be administered to infants at 4-month intervals. The questionnaires were composed of items that asked parents or other caregivers simple questions about their infant's behavior. Once completed, the questionnaires were mailed back to a central site for scoring. It was imperative to examine the questionnaires' validity and reliability because, during the 1970s and well into the 1980s, many professionals were highly skeptical of parental ability to accurately assess their child's development.

In 1980, we received a grant from the National Institute on Handicapped Research, U.S. Office of Education.[2] The major goal of this project was to establish a monitoring system using the six parent-completed questionnaires at 4-month intervals. Infants considered to be at risk for developmental delay were evaluated from 4 to 24 months of age. Related objectives included 1) comparing the accuracy of the parental monitoring with an evaluation completed by a professional, and 2) determining whether there were factors (e.g., level of education) that predicted the type of parent who can accurately complete the questionnaires. The findings from this 3-year study were extremely encouraging. First, we found that most parents had no trouble understanding and completing the questionnaires. Second, the test–retest and interrater reliability were more than 90%. Finally, there was strong agreement between parents' classification of their infant using the questionnaires and a trained examiner's classification using the Revised Gesell Developmental Examination (Knobloch et al., 1980). Modest overreferral for further evaluation occurred, while more substantial underreferral occurred. These findings were promising enough to suggest the questionnaires should receive further study.

From 1983 to 1985, work continued on the questionnaires largely through the monitoring of infants discharged from the neonatal intensive care unit of our regional medical facility, Sacred Heart General Hospital. It was during this time that the original six questionnaires were refined and questionnaires targeting children 30 and 36 months of age were developed. In 1985, a grant was received from the National Institute on Disability and Rehabilitation Research, U.S. Office of Education. The objectives of this 3-year project were to examine 1) agreement between parental classification and trained examiners' classification—specifically examining overreferral, underreferral, sensitivity, and specificity; 2) test–retest and interrater reliability; and 3) cost of using the questionnaires. In general, project results supported previous findings. The agreement between parents and professionals on the classification of the infant or child was generally high, although variations occurred across intervals. Underreferral was low, while overreferral varied considerably across age intervals but was generally acceptable. Specificity was high, while sensitivity varied from low to moderate, suggesting some change in questionnaire scoring was in order. Reliability continued to be high, and the cost of using the questionnaires was found to be modest—approximately $2.50 for each questionnaire.

In 1988, we received a 2-year Social and Behavioral Sciences Research Grant from the March of Dimes Research Foundation, and in 1990, a 2-year continuation was granted. The subjects addressed by this project included 1) examining the use of the questionnaires with a group of low-income parents, and 2) assessing the effect of completing the questionnaires on parents' attitudes and knowledge of development. Results from this project suggested that low-income parents and caregivers with limited education can successfully and accurately complete the *Ages & Stages Questionnaires*; however,

[2]Now the U.S. Office of Education, National Institute on Disability and Rehabilitation Research.

the relatively small sample required caution in generalizing these findings to broad groups of parents. We did not find that completion of the questionnaires produced measurable effects on parents' attitudes or knowledge of development. Interestingly, this latter finding was in conflict with feedback we were receiving from the field. Many parents and practitioners who were using the questionnaires insisted the questionnaires assisted them in observing, understanding, and teaching their infant or young child.

Collection of data on the questionnaires from the early 1980s permitted assembling a database including both children developing typically and children at risk. This database was used to make revisions on the questionnaires in 1990–1991. The data analyses suggested only minor changes were necessary. A questionnaire targeting 48-month-old children was developed in 1992, and supplemental questionnaires for 6 and 18 months were developed. In 1997–1998, the 60 month questionnaire was developed and tested. Alternate form questionnaires for 10, 14, 22, 27, 33, 42, and 54 months were completed.

Another grant to study the questionnaires was received in 1991, again from the National Institute on Disability and Rehabilitation Research. This project was designed to help expand questions addressed by the previous March of Dimes–supported project, specifically 1) Can parents from extremely high-risk populations accurately complete the questionnaires? and 2) Does completion of the questionnaires affect parents' attitudes and knowledge of early development? Results from this 3-year project largely replicated and expanded our earlier findings. Parents with extremely low incomes, parents with limited educational backgrounds, teenage parents, and parents who abused substances served as subjects. These parents were able to accurately complete questionnaires on their infants and young children (Squires, Potter, Bricker, & Lamorey, 1998). Although the findings for the question on parents' attitudes and knowledge of early development were complex, in large measure we found that completion of the questionnaires did not result in significant attitude change or enhanced knowledge of development.

In addition to our empirical work, we have received constructive feedback on the questionnaires from parents, early intervention program personnel, and professionals who use the ASQ to monitor infants and young children. The questionnaires are being used in a large number of local agencies, regional programs, and statewide monitoring systems. Project staff have shared a variety of information and data with us. When possible, the data have been combined with our existing data sets and included in analyses to improve the generalizability of the results. Feedback on questionnaire format and monitoring procedures have been incorporated into the ASQ system as appropriate. We are extremely grateful for the feedback that has, we believe, improved the questionnaires.

Findings on the questionnaires have been extensively published. This list of publications is included in Appendix A of this volume. A description of all data analyses and results are contained in Appendix F. As Appendix F indicates, much time and effort have been expended to examine the questionnaires. Although further work remains to be done, we believe that the current database indicates that the validity and reliability of the questionnaires were adequate to warrant their release for publication.

Based on almost 20 years of research findings, the first edition of the *Ages & Stages Questionnaires* was published in 1995. Commercial publishing and increased distribution of the ASQ has allowed a wide variety of education, health, and social services agencies to screen and monitor young children for developmental problems. Home visiting programs such as Healthy Start and

Parents as Teachers; public health nursing programs in New York and southwest Minnesota; and Child Find efforts in Idaho, North Dakota, Florida, and Hawaii have made the ASQ an integral program component. Pediatricians, nurses, social welfare workers, and early intervention screening teams have successfully used and endorsed the ASQ as a cost-effective measure for identifying developmental delays in young children (see, e.g., Dworkin & Glascoe, 1997).

With expanded use of the ASQ and continued feedback from the field, two requests were made to us repeatedly. The first request was to extend the ASQ intervals to encompass the entire preschool span from 4 months to 5 years. The second request was to add questionnaires to fill in the age intervals so that children of any age could be screened.

In 1996, we began acting on the first request by writing and developing the 60 month questionnaire. Developmental resources such as standardized and curriculum-based assessments and kindergarten curricula were used as the basis for the 60 month questionnaire items. After field-testing two editions of this questionnaire between 1996 and 1998, a final version of the 60 month questionnaire was completed, and concurrent validity and reliability studies were undertaken in early 1998.

In 1997, work was begun on the second request. Supplemental questionnaires to address missing age intervals (e.g., 10 months) were created and field-tested to develop an ASQ system that could accommodate children of any age between 4 months and 60 months. Like the 6 and 18 month questionnaires, these supplemental questionnaires were composed of empirically tested items that were taken from the ASQ questionnaires at 4, 8, 12, 16, 20, 24, 30, 36, and 48 months. Supplemental questionnaires at 6, 10, 14, 18, 22, 27, 33, 42, and 54 months filled out the series for a total of 19 questionnaires. Data collection on the 60 month and supplemental questionnaires is ongoing.

This second edition of the ASQ includes the original questionnaire intervals of 4, 8, 12, 16, 20, 24, 30, 36, and 48 months as well as the newly developed 60 month interval. In addition, the second edition contains copies of the 9 supplemental questionnaires at 6, 10, 14, 18, 22, 27, 33, 42, and 54 months. This *User's Guide* has been updated when necessary. We are hopeful that the expansion of the ASQ system contained in this second edition will make this tool increasingly attractive and useful to programs and personnel interested in screening and tracking young children during their early years of life.

Also in 1997, with the passage of the amendments to the Individuals with Disabilities Education Act (IDEA), came a call for early detection of social or emotional problems in young children. In response to this urgent need, we have developed the *Ages & Stages Questionnaires: Social-Emotional*—available in both English and Spanish—and an accompanying *User's Guide*. This screening tool, meant to be used in conjunction with a general developmental tool (like the ASQ) that assesses cognitive, communicative, and motor development, helps identify the need for further social and emotional behavior assessment in children at eight age intervals: 6, 12, 18, 24, 30, 36, 48, and 60 months. These eight ASQ:SE questionnaires each address seven behavioral areas: self-regulation, compliance, communication, adaptive functioning, autonomy, affect, and interaction with people.

We are hopeful that the increased availability of the *Ages & Stages Questionnaires* and *the Ages & Stages Questionnaires: Social-Emotional* will improve the screening and tracking efforts of programs throughout the United States and elsewhere. Photocopying is permitted according to the following guidelines:

Purchasers of the ***Ages & Stages Questionnaires®: A Parent-Completed, Child-Monitoring System*** *are granted permission to photocopy the questionnaires as well as the sample letters and forms in* ***The ASQ User's Guide for the Ages & Stages Questionnaires®: A Parent-Completed, Child-Monitoring System*** *in the course of their agency's service provision to families.* Each branch office that will be using the ASQ system must purchase its own set of original questionnaires; master forms cannot be shared among sites. The questionnaires and samples are meant to be used to facilitate screening and monitoring and to assist in the early identification of children who may need further evaluation. Electronic reproduction of the questionnaires is prohibited, and none of the ASQ materials may be reproduced to generate revenue for any program or individual. Photocopies may only be made from an original set of color-coded master questionnaires and/or an original ***User's Guide***. Programs are prohibited from charging parents, caregivers, or other service providers who will be completing and/or scoring the questionnaires fees in excess of the exact cost to photocopy the master forms. This restriction is not meant to apply to reimbursement of usual and customary charges for developmental screening when performed with other evaluation and management services. The ASQ materials may not be used in a way contrary to the family-oriented philosophies of the ASQ developers. *Unauthorized use beyond this privilege is prosecutable under federal law.* You will see the copyright protection line at the bottom of each form.

Improved screening programs should result in the efficient and accurate identification of infants and young children who will benefit from further evaluation and, if needed, timely intervention.

Diane Bricker, Ph.D.
Jane Squires, Ph.D.

REFERENCES

Bricker, D. (1996). The goal: Prediction or prevention? *Journal of Early Intervention, 20*(4), 294–296.

Dworkin, P.H., & Glascoe, F.P. (1997). Early detection of developmental delays: How do you measure up? *Contemporary Pediatrics, 14*(4), 158–168.

Hack, M., Breslau, N., Weismann, B., Aram, D., Klein, N., & Borawski, E. (1991). Effect of very low birth weight and subnormal head size on cognitive abilities at school age. *New England Journal of Medicine, 325*(4), 231–277.

Knobloch, H., Stevens, F., & Malone, A.F. (1980). *Manual of developmental diagnosis: The administration and interpretation of the Revised Gesell and Amatruda Developmental and Neurological Examination.* Houston, TX: Developmental Evaluation Materials, Inc.

Knobloch, H., Stevens, F., Malone, A.F., Ellison, P., & Risemburg, H. (1979). The validity of parental reporting of infant development. *Pediatrics, 63,* 873–878.

Parmelee, A.H., & Cohen, S.E. (1985). Neonatal follow-up services for infants at risk. In S. Harel & N.J. Anastasiow (Eds.), *The at-risk infant: Psycho/socio/medical aspects* (pp. 269–273). Baltimore: Paul H. Brookes Publishing Co.

Sameroff, A. (1981). Longitudinal studies of preterm infants: A review of chapters 17–20. In S. Friedman & M. Sigman (Eds.), *Preterm birth and psychological development* (pp. 387–393). New York: Academic Press.

Scott, K., & Masi, W. (1979). The outcome from and utility of registers of risk. In T. Field, A. Sostek, S. Goldberg, & H. Shuman (Eds.), *Infants born at risk* (pp. 485–496). Jamaica, NY: Spectrum Publications.

Squires, J., Potter, L., Bricker, D., & Lamorey, S. (1998). Parent-completed developmental questionnaires: Effectiveness with low and middle income parents. *Early Childhood Research Quarterly, 13*(2), 347–356.

Werner, E.E., & Smith, R.S. (1992). *Overcoming the odds: High risk children from birth to adulthood.* Ithaca, NY: Cornell University Press.

Widerstrom, A.H., & Nickel, R.E. (1997). Determinants of risk in infancy. In A.H. Widerstrom, B.A. Mowder, & S.R. Sandall, *Infant development and risk: An introduction* (2nd ed., pp. 61–87). Baltimore: Paul H. Brookes Publishing Co.

Acknowledgments

ASQ™

In the late 1970s, when we began to think about the need to develop a monitoring system for early detection of infants who might need intervention, we did not realize how our simple idea would persist and grow over the years. The idea—asking parents to monitor the development of their infants using easy-to-complete questionnaires—had immediate appeal to a range of parents and professionals and quickly took on a life of its own. Because of the questionnaires' instant appeal, caregivers and practitioners often saw no need to determine their psychometric properties and utility for a range of users. Over the years, we have been told repeatedly by an array of parents and professionals, "I know they [the questionnaires] work. Why do you need to conduct studies?" In spite of their instantaneous acceptance and strong face validity, we felt obligated to assess the validity, reliability, and utility of the *Ages & Stages Questionnaires* (ASQ), then called the Infant/Child Monitoring Questionnaires, across a range of children and families. We have been addressing this challenge since 1980. Although work remains to be done, we now feel comfortable with the questionnaires' use in identifying with relative accuracy infants and young children who need further assessment. As with any screening tool, some under- and overreferral occurs. The dynamic nature of development and errors inherent in measurement probably make the creation of an ideal tool impossible; however, we believe the *Ages & Stages Questionnaires* offers one of the better screening options available.

In 1979, Hilda Knobloch and her colleagues published an article describing parental ability to report on their infant's development. Dr. Knobloch's approach served as the inspiration for the development of the ASQ system. We are grateful to Laurel Carlson for directing our attention to this article.

Support from the U.S. Department of Education and the March of Dimes Research Foundation has permitted almost continuous empirical study of the questionnaires since 1980. The early work was largely conducted on infants recruited from Sacred Heart General Hospital located in Eugene, Oregon. Support and assistance from the hospital's research committee and neonatal intensive care unit (NICU) were extremely important. Laurel Carlson and Robert Nickel were largely responsible for developing the lines of communication with the hospital's NICU and the local pediatric community that permitted us to conduct our early work.

Over the 18-year span of projects associated with the ASQ system, many individuals assisted in planning and conducting data collection efforts. In particular, we would like to acknowledge Linda Mounts for her many contributions to the project, Ann Marie Jusczyk for her help in recruiting and testing subjects, and Suzanne Lamorey for coordinating data collection activities for the National Institute on Disability and Rehabilitation Research project. In addition, we would like to thank Doris Potter for contributing her photographs to this *User's Guide.*

Thousands of infants and children and their families have completed and returned questionnaires, and many have been willing to participate in a range of testing with a variety of instruments. Without the data generated by these children and their parents, we would have been unable to examine the reliability, validity, and utility of the questionnaires.

In addition to parents and children, we have received valuable feedback about the questionnaires from professionals who are using them. In particular, we thank the Hawaii Planning Team: Ginger Fink, Kamehameha Schools; Ruth Ota, Public Health Nursing Branch; Patsy Murakami, Preschool Screening Program; Roma Johnson, 0–3 Hawaii Project; Gladys Wong, Maternal and Child Health Branch; and Shair Neilson, Center on the Family, for suggesting questionnaire format changes that improved ease of use and appeal to parents.

The success of any complex long-term project is dependent upon an array of factors, including consistent financial support, commitment from project staff, subjects' good faith participation, ideas with merit, reasonable and practical plans of action, and luck. We have been fortunate to have had all of these.

Diane Bricker, Ph.D.
Jane Squires, Ph.D.
December, 1998

THE ASQ USER'S GUIDE
SECOND EDITION

ASQ™

I Overview of ASQ

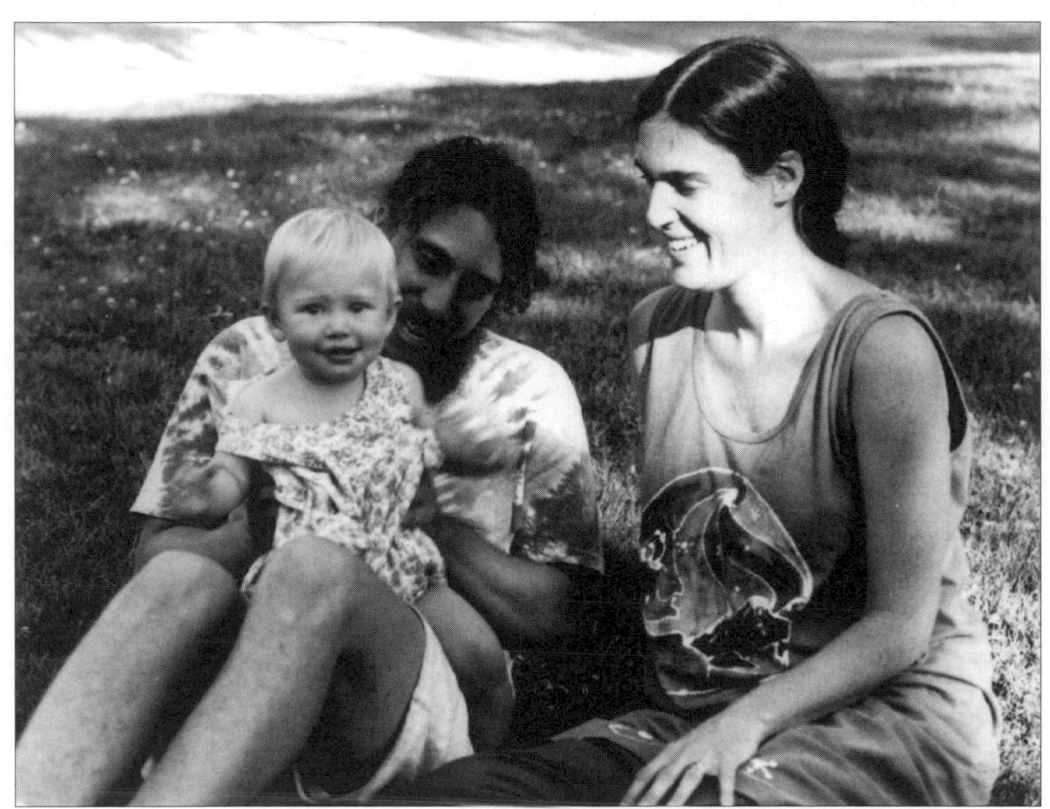

1 Introduction to ASQ

A major obstacle to the timely delivery of early intervention services is the early and accurate identification of infants and young children who have developmental delays or disorders. The first step in obtaining needed services for infants and young children and their families is the establishment of comprehensive, first-level screening programs. The goal of comprehensive Child Find programs is to separate accurately the few infants and young children who require more extensive evaluation from the children who do not. To be useful, first-level screening programs need to assess large numbers of children and, therefore, require screening measures or procedures that are easy to administer, at a low cost, and appropriate for diverse populations. The *Ages & Stages Questionnaires (ASQ): A Parent-Completed, Child-Monitoring System, Second Edition,* meets these criteria for a first-level comprehensive screening program. The ASQ screening system is composed of 19 questionnaires designed to be completed by parents[1] or primary caregivers. Questionnaire intervals include 4, 6, 8, 10, 12, 14, 16, 18, 20, 22, 24, 27, 30, 33, 36, 42, 48, 54, and 60 months of age. In most cases, these questionnaires can identify accurately infants or young children who are in need of further evaluation to determine whether they are eligible for early intervention services.

Each questionnaire contains 30 developmental items that are written in simple, straightforward language. The items are divided into five areas: communication, gross motor, fine motor, problem solving, and personal-social. An Overall section addresses general parental concerns. The reading level of each questionnaire ranges from the fourth to the sixth grade. Illustrations are provided when possible to assist parents and caregivers in understanding the items. For the 30 developmental items, parents check *yes* to indicate that their child performs the behavior specified in the item, *sometimes* to indicate an occasional or emerging response from their child, or *not yet* to indicate that their child does not yet perform the behavior. Program staff convert each response to a point value, total these values, and compare the total score to established screening cutoff points.

[1]Throughout this book and in the *Ages & Stages Questionnaires* themselves, "parents" is used to refer to individuals central to a child's life, including parents, grandparents, and other primary caregivers.

ASQ MATERIALS

The ASQ materials consist of 19 photocopiable master questionnaires; 19 photocopiable, age-appropriate scoring and data summary sheets; and this *User's Guide.* The master set of questionnaires allows program personnel to select age intervals and reproduce the necessary number of copies, depending on the participating children and families. Spanish and French translations of the questionnaires are also available. This *User's Guide* contains vital information about planning, using, and evaluating the monitoring system as well as summary information on the psychometric studies conducted on the ASQ system. Instructions for scoring questionnaires; sample letters to parents, agencies, and service providers; and activities sheets for parents that correspond to the ASQ age intervals are also included in this *User's Guide.* A supplementary videotape, *The Ages & Stages Questionnaires on a Home Visit* (Farrell & Potter, 1995), describes procedures for using the questionnaires while conducting home visits. The ASQ Manager software enables users to create a database for managing and tracking ASQ data for many children. The *Ages & Stages Questionnaires: Social-Emotional* (ASQ:SE) takes the ASQ a step further by concentrating on the importance of considering social and emotional competence in young children at eight stages. The *ASQ:SE* contains 8 reproducible master questionnaires and 8 reproducible, age-appropriate scoring and data summary sheets. A Spanish translation of the ASQ:SE questionnaires is also available. *The ASQ:SE User's Guide* describes variables for assessment; explains how to contend with the differences in time and setting, development, individual, and family/culture that may affect results; and offers strategies for using the ASQ:SE. The ASQ and ASQ:SE questionnaires (plus intervention activities) are also available in CD-ROM format (in English or Spanish). Two additional videos, *ASQ Scoring and Referral* and *ASQ:SE in Practice,* are now available.

USING THE ASQ SYSTEM

The questionnaires can be used for two important purposes. First, they can be used for comprehensive, first-level screening of large groups of infants and young children. For example, parents can complete questionnaires on their child prior to a kindergarten roundup or at well-baby checkups. Second, the questionnaires can be used to monitor the development of children who are at risk for developmental disabilities or delays resulting from medical factors such as low birth weight, prematurity, seizures, serious illness or from environmental factors such as poverty, parents with mental impairments, history of abuse and/or neglect in the home, or teenage parents.

Use of the questionnaires is flexible for either first-level screening or monitoring programs. For example, questionnaires can be used at 6-month intervals, one time only (e.g., 12 months), or at a few selected intervals (e.g., 12, 24, and 33 months).

The questionnaires are designed to be completed by the child's parents or caregivers in the home. Questionnaires can be mailed to parents or caregivers, who can then try each activity with the child and observe whether he or she can perform the designated behaviors. Questionnaires are then returned by mail to a central location for scoring or brought to a primary care clinic for scoring and discussion during a well-child examination. Alternatively, questionnaires can be completed during home visits with the assistance of service providers. In addition, questionnaires can be completed in waiting rooms, clinics, schools, and child care environments by parents or other caregivers.

ADMINISTRATION AND SCORING

Each questionnaire can be completed in 10–15 minutes. Scoring can be done by clerical staff or paraprofessionals who have been instructed by professional staff; scoring can take as little as 1 minute and no more than 5 minutes. An ASQ Information Summary Sheet is included for each age interval. This form provides space for scoring the questionnaire as well as space to record demographic information about the family and overall comments of the parents or caregivers. This sheet permits professional staff to keep a one-page summary of questionnaire results while allowing parents to keep the questionnaire for further reference about their child's developmental level.

To score a questionnaire, the parents' responses—*yes, sometimes,* and *not yet*—are converted to points—*10, 5,* and *0,* respectively—and are totaled for each area. These five area scores are then compared with empirically derived cutoff points that are shown on bar graphs on the ASQ Information Summary Sheets. If the child's score falls in the shaded portion of the bar graph in any developmental area (e.g., fine motor, communication), then further diagnostic assessment is recommended.

Although the questionnaires are designed to be completed by parents, the system requires professional involvement. One or more professionals will be needed to establish the system, develop the necessary community interfaces, train individuals who will score the questionnaires, and provide feedback to parents of children who are completing the questionnaires. Paraprofessionals can operate the system once it is established, score the questionnaires, and provide routine feedback to families of children who are not identified as requiring further assessment.

RESEARCH ON THE ASQ SYSTEM

Study of the ASQ began in 1980 when it was first called the Infant/Child Monitoring Questionnaires. Since 1980, a number of investigations have examined the validity, reliability, and utility of the ASQ. To examine the validity of the ASQ, children's classifications on parent-completed questionnaires were compared with their classifications on professionally administered standardized assessments, including the Revised Gesell and Amatruda Developmental and Neurological Examination (Knobloch, Stevens, & Malone, 1980), the Bayley Scales of Infant Development (Bayley, 1969), the Stanford-Binet Intelligence Scale (Thorndike, Hagen, & Sattler, 1985), the McCarthy Scales of Children's Abilities (McCarthy, 1972), and the Battelle Developmental Inventory (Newborg, Stock, Wnek, Guidubaldi, & Svinicki, 1987). Overall agreement on children's classifications was 83%, with a range of 76%–91%. Sensitivity, specificity, underreferral and overreferral rates, and positive predictive values are reported in Appendix F of this book.

Studies on the reliability of the questionnaires have examined interrater and test–retest reliability as well as internal consistency. Test–retest information was collected by asking a group of 175 parents to complete two questionnaires on their children at 2- to 3-week intervals. Classification of each child based on the parents' scoring of the two questionnaires was compared and was found to exceed 90% agreement. Interrater reliability was assessed by having a trained examiner complete a questionnaire on a child shortly after the parent had completed one. Overall agreement on the classification of the

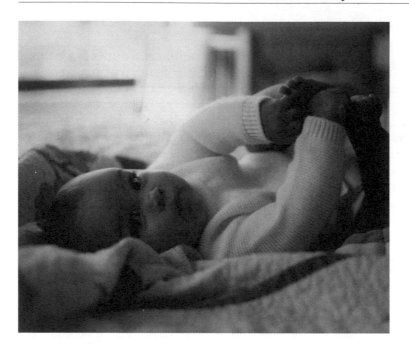

child among 112 parents and 3 trained examiners exceeded 90%. These and other reliability data are discussed in Appendix F of this book.

ADVANTAGES OF THE ASQ SYSTEM

Assessments of infants and young children should be done on a regular and periodic basis because of the rapid developmental changes in the early years (Meisels & Provence, 1989; Squires, Nickel, & Eisert, 1996). Because professional assessments are expensive and are usually not performed at regular intervals, the use of more cost-effective means (e.g., parent-completed tools) may be better suited for the periodic monitoring of early development.

The ASQ system relies on parents to observe their child and to complete the simple questionnaires about their child's abilities. In addition to being cost-effective, using parents to complete developmental questionnaires may enhance the accuracy of screening assessments because of the variety and array of information parents have about their children (Clark, Paulson, & Conlin, 1993). Another advantage is that using parent-completed tools such as ASQ fulfills the spirit of the Individuals with Disabilities Education Act Amendments of 1997 (PL 105-17), which call for parents to be partners in their child's assessment and intervention activities.

A final advantage is the flexibility of the ASQ system. The ASQ system can be adapted to a variety of environments, including the home, primary care clinics, child care environments, preschool programs, and teen parenting programs. Questionnaires may be completed by parents during home visits from nurses, social workers, or paraprofessionals.

Using the master set, screening programs may choose ASQ age intervals that fit their populations, program goals, and needs. For example, medical practitioners may use the 6 month ASQ interval because it corresponds to the time of well-child visits. Public health home visiting programs may choose the 4 and 8 month ASQ age intervals because they correspond to home visiting schedules. Head Start programs may use only the 48 month questionnaire, and toddler programs may choose to use the 12, 14, 16, 18, 20, 22, 24, 27, and 30 month questionnaires. The ASQ system is flexible and can fit the needs of diverse monitoring and screening programs.

HOW TO USE THIS GUIDE

This *User's Guide* is written for professionals and paraprofessionals who plan to use the ASQ system. The remaining chapters provide information on the background and use of the ASQ system and step-by-step instructions for planning, using, and evaluating the monitoring system. Chapter 2 focuses on the need for screening and monitoring, previous approaches to screening, problems with these approaches, and the inception and development of the ASQ system. Chapter 3 describes in detail the materials and phases of the ASQ system. Chapters 4–6 describe the implementation of the ASQ system. Instructions and detailed figures are intended to guide readers through the phases, while a program case study illustrates the process. This volume's glossary is intended as a helpful reference while both planning and implementing the monitoring program. The appendices provide valuable supplemental information, including a summary of the validity and reliability research conducted on the ASQ system.

2

The Need for ASQ

ASQ™

Most people believe that the quality of life experienced during infancy and young childhood has a significant effect on subsequent development. Serious medical, biological, or environmental problems demand swift attention and remediation if maximum development is to be attained. Therefore, early identification of children whose developmental trajectory is delayed or atypical is essential in order to institute timely action to correct or attenuate problems. Early identification of children with developmental or behavior problems is predicated on the assumption that a distinction is possible between children whose development is uneventful or whose problems are transitory and children who are facing serious and persistent developmental challenges. Steady progress has been made toward the timely identification of children with disabilities during the 20th century.

NEED FOR SCREENING AND MONITORING

In addition to a general societal consensus that early detection of problems is a worthwhile goal, other important factors have contributed to the growing commitment by local, state, and federally funded agencies to monitor the development of designated groups of infants and young children. These factors include

- A growing population of infants at risk for developmental disabilities because of environmental conditions such as poverty and neglect
- Increased emphasis on prevention of developmental disabilities and chronic illnesses
- Federal and state legal and statutory regulations addressing the need for early and effective Child Find programs

These factors have led to a growing number of federal- and state-supported programs designed to identify and track the development of infants and young children who are at risk for future problems. This growth in early identification and monitoring of risk groups has resulted in a need for reliable and cost-effective approaches for screening and Child Find programs. To be effective, tests and procedures must accurately discriminate between children who require further assessment and those who do not. To conduct comprehensive evaluations of children who have no problems or children whose problems are transitory is a poor use of limited resources. To overlook children who have problems that are likely to persist or become serious is wasteful for the children, their families, and the community.

The need for effective screening and monitoring of infants and young children considered at risk for developmental disabilities and the lack of low-cost strategies was the impetus for the development of the *Ages & Stages Questionnaires* (ASQ). To provide a context for the ASQ approach, other screening and monitoring procedures are reviewed.

SCREENING AND MONITORING APPROACHES

Screening and monitoring of infants and young children have been conducted primarily by means of periodic follow-up with designated groups of infants considered to be at risk for developmental disabilities. The major exception to this basic approach has been the general screening procedures conducted in the public schools with children entering kindergarten or first grade. Most screening programs conducted with infants have focused on populations who are at risk for developmental disabilities as a result of medical, biological, or environmental circumstances (Meisels & Provence, 1989). Screening approaches can be classified as four types: the multidisciplinary team approach, the well-baby checkups approach, the community-based evaluation "round up" approach, and the parent monitoring approach.

Multidisciplinary Team Approach

A prevalent approach, in vogue beginning in the 1970s and throughout the 1980s and 1990s, is the multidisciplinary team assessment of designated groups of infants at risk for developmental disabilities. An example of this type of approach is the screening at preestablished intervals of groups of premature infants with low birth weights who meet specific criteria (e.g., Mitchell, Bee, Hammond, & Barnard, 1985). Much of the screening conducted by multidisciplinary teams was designed to determine the frequency of problems in specific populations of infants and/or to locate predictor variables. Using this approach, infants are brought to evaluation centers at established intervals and are assessed with one or more standardized measures by highly trained professionals. Often the children are given medical or neurological examinations as well.

Well-Baby Checkups Approach

A second approach to screening and monitoring is to identify infants and young children at well-baby checkups in physicians' offices or in public health facilities. Tests such as the Denver Developmental Screening Test (Frankenburg & Dodds, 1970) and the Revised Developmental Screening Inventory (Knobloch et al., 1980) are used by professionals or other personnel to assess the developmental status of the infant or young child. These tests are quick to administer and can be used with infants and young children at any age.

Community-Based Evaluation "Round Up" Approach

A third approach is the community-based evaluation "round up." Round ups encourage parents to bring their infants or young children to an evaluation center for screening. These "round ups" can be held one to four times per year and are staffed by professionals and volunteers. Tools such as the Developmental Indicators for the Assessment of Learning–Revised (Mardell-Czudnowski & Goldenberg, 1983) and the Early Screening Inventory (Meisels & Wiske, 1982) are administered by professionals and other staff. Volunteers may assist in the assessment process, and the tools used are usually easy to administer and can be used efficiently with large groups of children.

Parent Monitoring Approach

Having parents monitor their children's development is a fourth approach to screening (Bricker & Squires, 1989; Squires et al., 1996; Squires & Bricker, 1991; Squires, Bricker, & Potter, 1997; Squires, Nickel, & Bricker, 1990). An example of a parent monitoring approach is the use of The Denver Prescreening Developmental Questionnaire (Frankenburg, Van Doorninck, Liddell, & Dick, 1976) in a physician's office. This tool is designed to be completed quickly by parents prior to medical or evaluation visits. Knobloch and her associates (Knobloch, Stevens, Malone, Ellison, & Risemburg, 1979) developed the Revised Parent Developmental Questionnaire for the same purpose. These measures require minimal professional input and can be used at any age. The *Ages & Stages Questionnaires* is another example of a parent monitoring approach. Although the ASQ system shares similarities with each of the tests previously discussed, the ASQ system also differs in important ways.

SCREENING AND MONITORING CHALLENGES

Perhaps the first and most important challenge for the timely identification of problems in infants and young children is the dynamic nature of development. Development in most children proceeds at a predictable rate and in a predictable fashion. That is, most children learn to roll over before they crawl and pull to stand before they walk; however, within such developmental sequences, extensive variations can occur for a variety of reasons. Sometimes these variations do not cause concern (e.g., some children never learn to crawl but do learn to walk without problem), whereas other variations can lead to increasingly serious problems. Developmental variations do not occur at specified times. That is, children may develop difficulties at any point in time. For example, if a medical problem occurs when the child is 9 months old, the condition may have a brief or a lasting effect on the child's subsequent development. In addition, infants raised in poverty may not show developmental aberrations until 2 or 3 years of age, or they may show none at all. Because the nature of physiological or environmental conditions confronting individual children cannot be reliably predicted over time, one cannot assume that because a child's developmental trajectory is on target at 9 months, it will remain on target over time. In addition, one should not assume that an infant developing poorly at 4 months will continue to develop poorly over time.

Because of the dynamic nature of development, children should be screened systematically over time. Screening programs that assess children at only one point in time will likely overlook children whose development problems occur after the assessment interval. In addition, if the screening occurs initially at 4 or 5 years, then timely identification of problems may be delayed by, literally, years. Programs that screen children repeatedly but at infrequent intervals also run the risk of not detecting problems in children

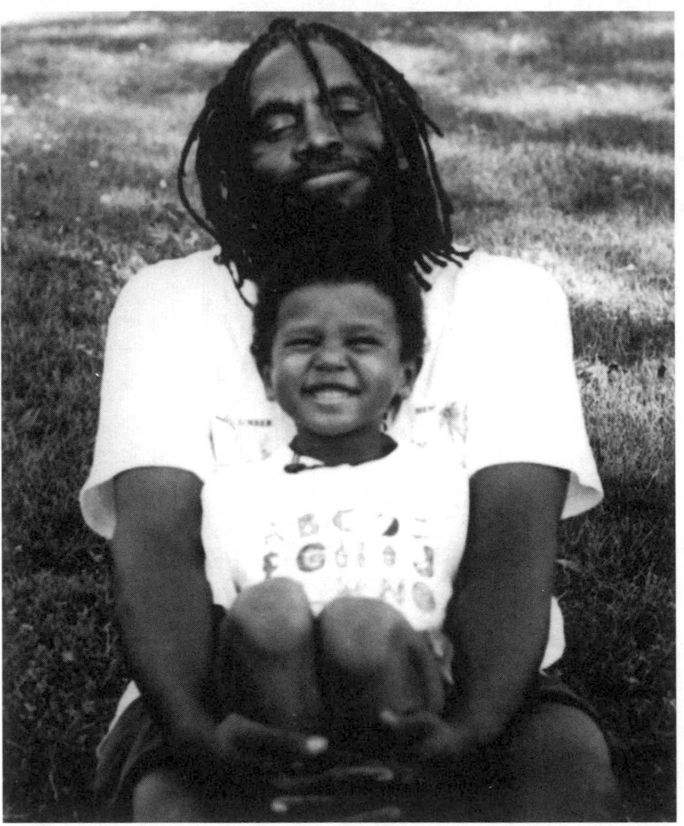

in a timely manner. Effective programs screen children at frequent intervals; however, frequent screening dictates the use of economical procedures to keep costs low.

A second challenge for screening and monitoring programs is to include parents in the assessment of their children's developmental status. Screening and monitoring measures that are completed by professionals with minimal parental input do not reflect the intent of U.S. federal law or recommended practices in early intervention. Beginning with the Education of the Handicapped Act Amendments of 1983 (PL 98-199), then with the Education of the Handicapped Act Amendments of 1986 (PL 99-457), and finally with the Individuals with Disabilities Education Act Amendments of 1997 (PL 105-17), federal legislation has made it increasingly clear that parents have the right and should be encouraged to become involved in their child's assessment, intervention, and evaluation (Squires et al., 1996). The use of screening systems that do not include parents in meaningful and useful ways disregards this important mandate. In addition, recommended practice dictates the involvement of families to ensure that the rich, extensive reservoir of information that parents and other caregivers hold about the child is tapped. Failure to gather and use parental information for determining the child's developmental status results in, at best, an incomplete assessment picture. Inclusion of families in child assessment activities is also a recommended practice because that involvement has the potential to assist parents in acquiring critical information concerning their child as well as to develop more appropriate developmental expectations for their child.

A third challenge for screening and monitoring approaches is cost. Screening and monitoring large groups of children is expensive. When approaches employ the use of highly skilled professionals to conduct the screening procedure with designated target populations, the cost of frequent screening becomes prohibitive, which likely explains the reason that most of these programs screen children only once or at infrequent intervals. The cost of detecting the small number of children in need of follow-up can be very high for approaches that rely on skilled professionals, given that most children's development proceeds as expected. Many investigators indicate that only 30% of the children in their at-risk monitoring groups required intervention services by school age (Bricker, Squires, Kaminski, & Mounts, 1988). For example, if a group of 100 children are screened once per year for 6 years at the moderate cost of $50 per assessment, the total cost for screening all of the children is $30,000, or $300 per child. A first-level screening approach that employs parents to complete developmental questionnaires can help keep the cost of screening and monitoring large groups of children in line with the program's existing resources.

THE AGES & STAGES QUESTIONNAIRES

The *Ages & Stages Questionnaires* (ASQ), initially called the Infant/Child Monitoring Questionnaires, were specifically developed to address the challenges described in the previous section. The ASQ system addresses the dynamic nature of development by offering multiple assessment intervals. Inclusion of parents is ensured either by having parents actually complete the questionnaires or by having program staff assist parents. The need for cost accountability is addressed by using parents to monitor their children's developmental progress.

The ASQ system has three components: 1) a set of questionnaires, 2) procedures for efficient and effective use of the questionnaires, and 3) support materials for use with the questionnaires. The ASQ system can be implemented in three phases: 1) planning the monitoring program, 2) using and scoring the questionnaires, and 3) evaluating the monitoring program.

ADVANTAGES AND LIMITATIONS OF THE ASQ SYSTEM

The primary advantage of using the ASQ system is that it is designed to assist parents in monitoring the development of their children. This feature allows enormous flexibility in the application and implementation of the system. The diverse goals of programs that screen and track children require a system that can adapt to the needs of a variety of families. By involving parents in the reporting of their children's developmental progress, a program has more flexibility in information gathering; this, of course, is affected by the commitment and abilities of the parents. The ASQ system's involvement of parents not only makes economic sense but also meets the mandates of the Individuals with Disabilities Education Act (IDEA) of 1990 (PL 101-476) and its 1997 amendments (PL 105-17), including—with the use of the ASQ:SE—the mandate for early detection of social or emotional problems in young children. Flexibility is built into completing, scoring, and implementing the ASQ system.

Completing the questionnaires is relatively simple and straightforward; therefore, it can be reliably accomplished by individuals with no specific training. Most motivated parents or other caregivers can complete the questionnaires without assistance, although some parents may require minimal assistance (e.g., help in interpreting some items). A few parents (e.g., those with mental health problems, those who cannot read) will need substantial assistance from a professional or paraprofessional in order to complete the questionnaires. The ASQ permits this type of flexibility in completion of individual questionnaires so that programs and professional staff can individualize their approach to diverse families.

Scoring a completed ASQ is also simple and straightforward and can be accomplished by a clerical worker or a paraprofessional. Item scores for each area are added and then compared to cutoff points provided on the last page of each questionnaire.

Creating a screening or monitoring system for using the questionnaires also can be adapted to meet the individual needs of communities, programs, and families. The questionnaires can be mailed to the child's home or completed during home visits; completed during a parent and child visit to an evaluation center, a well-baby checkup, or a physician's office; or completed during telephone interviews with the parents. Some communities and programs may choose to combine strategies so that most parents receive questionnaires through the mail while a few parents (e.g., those who cannot read) complete questionnaires through telephone interviews. Some communities may develop a system in which all physicians and medical clinics ask parents to complete questionnaires prior to their child's visit.

As with all screening systems, the ASQ has some limitations. First, some programs may need to assess infants or children at intervals not covered by the ASQ (e.g., 1 or 2 months of age). After the 36 month questionnaire, the time interval between questionnaires is 6 months (i.e., 42, 48, 54, and 60 month questionnaires). These 6-month intervals may prove to be problematic for programs that want to assess children between the specified questionnaire intervals (e.g., at 45 or 50 months). Second, using the ASQ requires an organizational structure that ensures parents are receiving and returning questionnaires as directed by the program. Systems need to be in place and monitored to check that questionnaires are mailed or given to parents and that information is collected (e.g., parents are interviewed) at the specified interval, that questionnaires are returned and appropriately scored, and that parents are given the necessary feedback. When screening large groups of children, procedures should be in place to ensure that the approach is implemented as planned. Finally, the ASQ will not be appropriate for use with all families. Some parents may be unwilling or unmotivated to complete questionnaires about their child, and some parents may find it offensive to complete the questionnaires. There are families that are in so much chaos that they are unable to comply. Parents who have mental or emotional impairments may be unable to understand the use of the questionnaires. For these parents and families, alternatives are necessary.

CONCLUSION

The heart of the ASQ system is parent or caregiver involvement. The pivotal role of parents in the ASQ system addresses the IDEA mandate of meaningful family inclusion. Inclusion of parents has the added feature of keeping screening costs within reason. In addition, flexibility in completing and scoring the questionnaires and implementing the ASQ system provide strong reasons to consider using the ASQ as a first-level screening approach. The components and phases of the ASQ system are described in Chapter 3.

3

The ASQ System

ASQ™

Screening and monitoring systems should accurately discriminate between infants and children who require further evaluation and those who do not. In addition, the screening and monitoring procedures should be kept at a low cost because large groups of children are involved. The ASQ system was developed to reliably identify children in need of further assessment and to do so at a low cost. The three components of the ASQ system—the questionnaires, the procedures for using and scoring the questionnaires, and the support materials that accompany the questionnaires—are described in this chapter. This chapter also describes the three phases of the ASQ system—planning the monitoring program, using and scoring the questionnaires, and evaluating the monitoring program.

COMPONENTS OF THE ASQ SYSTEM

Questionnaires

The ASQ system revolves around the use and scoring of its associated questionnaires. There are 19 questionnaires, which are designed to be administered at 4, 6, 8, 10, 12, 14, 16, 18, 20, 22, 24, 27, 30, 33, 36, 42, 48, 54, and 60 months. Each questionnaire contains simple questions addressing five specific developmental areas and one Overall section, which focuses on general parental concerns. Each questionnaire consists of the following elements:

- A title page that indicates the child's age, explains the questionnaires briefly, lists points to remember when completing the questionnaires, and provides a space for the program's identifying information
- An information sheet that asks for the child's name and other identifying information as well as who is completing the questionnaire
- Three or four pages with a total of 30 questions about the child's development, written in simple language and arranged hierarchically from easy to more difficult
- An Information Summary Sheet to be completed by the person scoring the questionnaire that includes a space for recording the child's identifying information, space for comments about the child's overall development,

scoring instructions, a grid that indicates developmental cutoff points, and an optional chart for recording responses to specific questionnaire items

Each questionnaire contains 30 questions, which are divided into the following five areas of development:

- *Communication,* which addresses babbling, vocalizing, listening, and understanding
- *Gross motor,* which focuses on arm, body, and leg movements
- *Fine motor,* which pertains to hand and finger movements
- *Problem solving,* which addresses learning and playing with toys
- *Personal-social,* which focuses on solitary social play and play with toys and other children

An *Overall* section asks about general parental concerns.

The questionnaire items were developed by examining the content of developmentally based, norm-referenced tests. Content that matched a specific test interval (e.g., 4, 8, 12 months) was used as the basis for the development of specific ASQ items. After the content was selected, a set of specific criteria was used to guide the writing of each questionnaire item. These criteria required that items 1) address important developmental milestones, 2) target behavior appropriate for the developmental quotient range of 75–100 for each age interval, 3) be easy for parents to observe and administer, and 4) use words that do not exceed a sixth-grade reading level. To further assist parents in using the questionnaires reliably, small illustrations are provided, where possible, beside the item to help convey the intent of the question. Figure 1 shows an item from the 16 month questionnaire. When relevant, written examples of the desired target behavior are included with the question. Throughout the questionnaires, male and female pronouns are alternated by item. The questionnaires are also available in Spanish, French, and Korean.

Ages & Stages Questionnaires—Spanish and French Versions All 19 of the questionnaires have been translated into Spanish and French and many of the form letters provided in this guide (see Appendix C) have been provided in Spanish. The Spanish questionnaires have been field tested with Spanish-speaking parents in a variety of geographic regions of the United States (e.g., Arizona, Texas, Washington); however, separate cutoff points have not been empirically derived as yet.

Ages & Stages Questionnaires: Social-Emotional The *Ages & Stages Questionnaires: Social-Emotional* is a screening tool, meant to be used in conjunction with the ASQ, to identify the need for further social and emotional behavior assessment in children from 6 to 60 months of age. Eight ques-

2. Does your child throw a small ball with a forward arm motion? (If she simply drops the ball, check "not yet" for this item.)

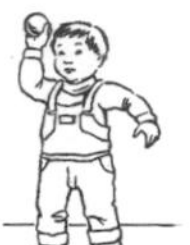

Figure 1. The questions on the *Ages & Stages Questionnaires*, like the one shown here, are straightforward and worded simply. Each of the questionnaires features 30 questions distributed evenly across five areas of development (communication, gross motor, fine motor, problem solving, and personal-social) and one Overall section designed to address parental concerns. Many are accompanied by illustrations to assist parents in evaluating their child's behavior and development.

tionnaires are available, in either English or Spanish, that address seven behavioral areas: Self-Regulation, Compliance, Communication, Adaptive Functioning, Autonomy, Affective, and Interaction with People. An accompanying *User's Guide* is also available to assist professionals in the effective use of the ASQ:SE questionnaires.

Psychometric Findings Data pertaining to both the validity and reliability of the ASQ system were collected over extended time periods with large numbers of children and families. These data are summarized next. For more detail, see Appendix F.

Questionnaire Validity The primary procedure used to examine the validity of the *Ages & Stages Questionnaires* has been to compare children's performance on the questionnaires with their performance on standardized developmental tests. Specifically, children's classifications based on parent-completed questionnaires were compared with the classifications derived from individually administered developmental tests by trained examiners. Comparisons for the 4 to 48 month questionnaires were made using the Revised Gesell and Amatruda Developmental and Neurological Examination (Knobloch et al., 1980), the Bayley Scales of Infant Development (Bayley, 1969), the Stanford-Binet Intelligence Scale (Thorndike et al., 1985), and the McCarthy Scales of Children's Abilities (McCarthy, 1972). Comparisons for the 60 month questionnaire were made using the Battelle Developmental Inventory (Newborg et al., 1987).

Validity data have been collected since 1981 using 1,763 assessments of infants and young children. Combined findings across years (see Appendix F) indicate that the overall agreement across questionnaires was 83%, with a range of 76%–91%. Underreferral (i.e., children not identified as having a developmental delay by the ASQ system who were diagnosed as having delays on the standardized assessment) across intervals ranged from 1% to 13%. Overscreening (i.e., children for whom the ASQ system indicated a delay who were categorized by the standardized assessment as developing typically) ranged from 7% to 16% across intervals. Sensitivity (i.e., children for whom the ASQ system indicated a delay and who were categorized by the standardized assessment as having a delay) ranged from 38% to 90%, and specificity (i.e., children for whom the ASQ system did not indicate a delay categorized by a standardized assessment as developing typically) ranged from 81% to 91%. Positive predictive value (i.e., a measure of the probability that a child with a questionnaire that indicated delay would have a poor outcome on the standardized assessment) ranged from 32% to 64%.

Questionnaire Reliability Test–retest and interrater reliability data have been collected for the ASQ system. Test–retest information was collected by asking a group of 175 parents to complete two questionnaires for their children at 2- to 3-week intervals. When completing the first questionnaire, the parents did not know that they would be asked to complete a second questionnaire. Classification of each child based on the parents' responses on the two questionnaires was compared and found to exceed 90% agreement.

Interrater reliability was assessed by having a trained examiner complete a questionnaire for a child shortly after a parent had completed a questionnaire. The parent was unaware of the comparison to be made, and the examiner had no knowledge of how the parent had responded on the questionnaire. Overall agreement on classification between 112 parents and 3 trained examiners was more than 90%.

ASQ Procedures for Using and Scoring Questionnaires

A variety of options can be considered for using the ASQ system. Frequently used options include mailing the questionnaires to the home, completing them on a home visit, and asking parents or service providers to complete them on site at a clinic or child care center. A combination of these options also can be used (e.g., giving the questionnaires to parents during a home visit and asking them to bring the questionnaires to their next well-child visit).

Several factors determine which options to use; each of these options is analyzed and outlined in detail in Chapter 5. First, resources must be considered. If personnel are available for home visits, then this may be the best option for some families, although this option will cost the monitoring program more than mailing the questionnaires to homes and asking families to return them by mail. Second, the characteristics of the families must be considered. Some families will need help to complete the questionnaires at home (e.g., parents with mental, physical, or emotional impairments). Home visits or on-site completion may need to be considered in cases like these. Third, preferences of families will be a factor in choosing which option to use. Some families may prefer completing the questionnaires with a home visitor during the day. Others may want to wait and complete the questionnaires when the working spouse is available in the evenings and then return them by mail. For some families, the options may change as life circumstances change.

Options for scoring the questionnaires are also available. The questionnaires may be scored by the monitoring program staff in their offices. Questionnaire results can then be given to parents by telephone, by mail, or on the next home visit. Alternately, staff can score the questionnaires on site or during a home visit and give parents immediate feedback. Because scoring takes only a few minutes, this can usually be done without delay. Parents can then keep the completed questionnaire while monitoring program staff can file the results recorded on the Information Summary Sheet. A last option is that parents themselves can score the questionnaires using the Information Summary Sheet. Again, options must be chosen based on parent preferences, family characteristics, and program resources.

ASQ Support Materials

In addition to this *User's Guide,* which contains complete instructions for each of the phases of the ASQ system and all of its components, numerous support materials accompany the *Ages & Stages Questionnaires.* Several of these materials are included in this guide:

- Sample forms to help with establishing the system (e.g., letters to parents, letters to physicians, demographic forms, evaluation forms)
- Guidelines for choosing referral criteria
- Supplemental materials, such as activities sheets that correspond to the ASQ age intervals
- ASQ technical report information (see Appendix F) that summarizes psychometric studies on the questionnaires (e.g., sample descriptions, analyses of reliability and validity, procedures for establishing cutoff points, comparisons of risk and nonrisk groups of children)

Information Summary Sheet Each *Ages & Stages Questionnaire* is accompanied by an Information Summary Sheet, which has the following two purposes: 1) to assist with scoring (see Chapter 5), and 2) to provide a summary of the child's performance on the questionnaire. The Information Summary Sheet can be kept by program staff as a record of the child's performance on the individual questionnaires so the questionnaires themselves can be returned to parents or service providers for future reference. The scoring section of the sheet is designed to be used primarily by service providers. Program staff can choose to use the entire Information Summary Sheet or only the scoring section, or they may choose not to use this form at all.

Additional Support Materials ASQ support materials sold separately include a CD-ROM in English or Spanish containing all of the ASQ questionnaires, plus the intervention activities sheets from the *User's Guide,* and videotapes that elaborate on ASQ and ASQ:SE home visits, questionnaire completion, scoring, and referral. On the videotape describing procedures for completing the ASQ with parents while on a home visit (Farrell & Potter, 1995), cultural adaptations, techniques for assisting parents to complete questionnaires, and suggestions for working in the home environment are enacted.

THREE PHASES OF THE ASQ SYSTEM

The ASQ system is composed of three phases, each of which is outlined next. Figure 2 provides an overview and relationship of the phases.

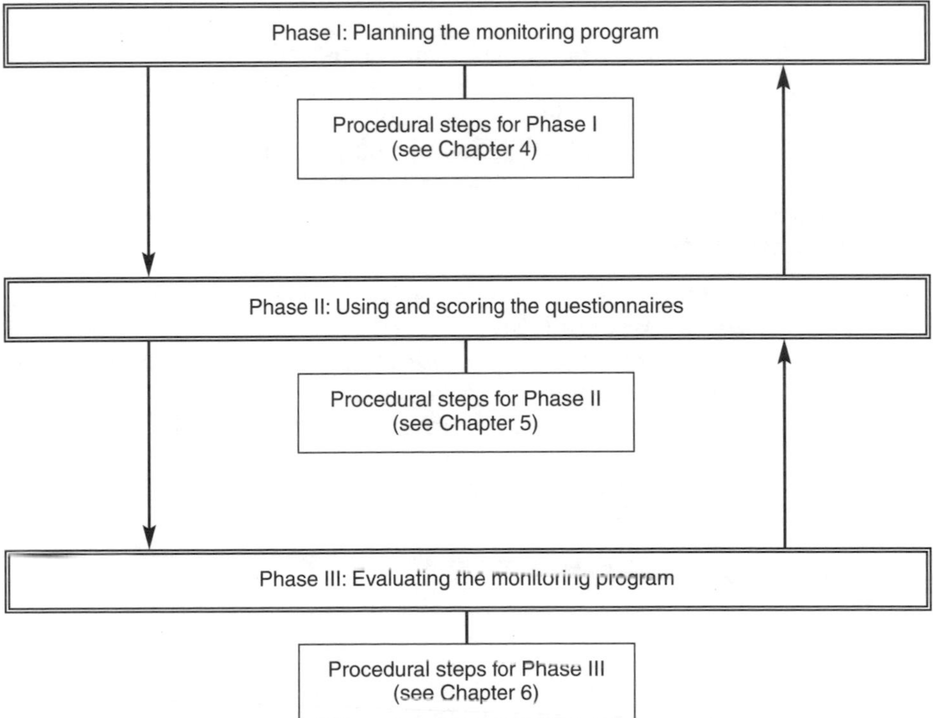

Figure 2. An overview of the ASQ system, focusing on its three interrelated phases: 1) planning the monitoring program, 2) using and scoring the questionnaires, and 3) evaluating the monitoring program. Each phase includes a number of steps to be performed before the phase is completed.

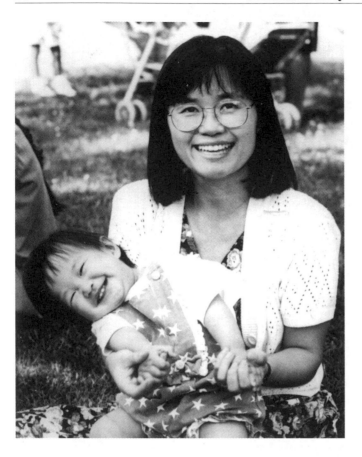

Planning the Monitoring Program

The first phase in the ASQ system is planning the monitoring program, which can involve the following seven steps:

1. Establish goals and objectives of the monitoring program.
2. Determine resources to conduct the monitoring program.
3. Determine method of using the questionnaires.
4. Select criteria for participation in the program.
5. Involve parents.
6. Involve physicians.
7. Outline referral criteria.

These steps, each of which is discussed in detail in Chapter 4, are suggested areas for consideration before beginning to use the questionnaires. Some programs may not need to devote planning time to all of the steps because agency policies may already address them. For example, program goals and objectives may already be delineated, and referral criteria may already be defined by state guidelines. Completing the planning phase helps to ensure that the monitoring system will run smoothly and efficiently once it is begun.

Using and Scoring the Questionnaires

The second phase of the ASQ system focuses on implementation—record keeping, step-by-step directions for scoring the questionnaires, and procedures for determining follow-up for children who are identified as needing further evaluation. This phase, which contains the details for day-to-day operation of the monitoring system, includes the following five steps:

1. Assemble child files.
2. Keep track of questionnaires.
3. Use the questionnaires.
4. Score the questionnaires.
5. Determine appropriate follow-up.

Chapter 5 outlines each of these steps and includes suggestions for maintaining child and family records and for establishing a tickler system.

Evaluating the Monitoring Program

The final phase of the ASQ system has two steps:

1. Assess progress in the establishment and maintenance of the monitoring program.
2. Evaluate the system's effectiveness.

Chapter 6 describes this final phase and includes a worksheet to guide evaluation of progress. Information helpful in measuring effectiveness, including how to calculate over- and underreferral rates and how to survey parents for feedback, is given. Completing evaluation activities on an ongoing basis helps to ensure that program procedures are efficient and that the monitoring system is effective—that is, that children in need of further diagnostic assessment are being identified.

CONCLUSION

This chapter describes the three components of the ASQ system—the questionnaires, the procedures for using and scoring the questionnaires, and the support materials. The heart of the ASQ system is the 19 child development questionnaires administered at regular intervals from 4 months to 60 months (5 years) of age. Support materials, including scoring guidelines and sample forms, assist with starting and maintaining the ASQ system. Information Summary Sheets are included with the *Ages & Stages Questionnaires.*

The three phases of establishing the ASQ system are also outlined in this chapter. Planning the monitoring program involves steps that are crucial to effective use of the ASQ system. The seven planning steps are described in detail in Chapter 4. Using and scoring the questionnaires, the second phase, focuses on implementation and includes record keeping, scoring directions, and procedures for determining follow-up for identified children. These steps are described in detail in Chapter 5. Finally, steps for the third phase, evaluation of the monitoring program, are discussed. A description of these two steps—assessing progress in the establishment and maintenance of the monitoring program, and evaluating the system's effectiveness—can be found in Chapter 6.

II Implementation of ASQ

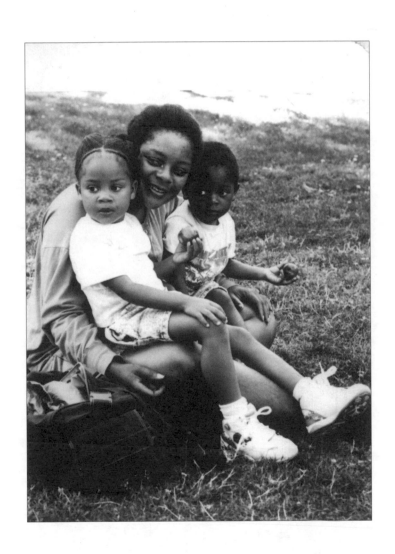

4

Phase I: Planning the Monitoring Program

ASQ™

A number of factors should be considered when initiating a screening and monitoring or Child Find program, such as the *Ages & Stages Questionnaires* system. This chapter describes each of the factors involved in the planning phase of the ASQ system.

IMPORTANCE OF THE PLANNING PHASE

The planning phase contains the most important steps toward establishing a successful monitoring program. Unless careful thought is given to each step at the beginning of the planning phase, serious difficulties may arise later when the program is in operation. For example, if community physicians and primary care practitioners are not consulted during this phase (see p. 39), referrals from physicians for children to participate in the monitoring program may be scarce. In addition, by involving physicians early in the program, more appropriate criteria for participation in the program (see pp. 32–34) and enhanced cooperation by physicians for completing health and developmental assessments may result. By spending adequate time during the planning phase, time and energy will be saved with smooth and effective program procedures.

STEPS IN THE PLANNING PHASE

Figure 3 provides a schematic of the factors, or steps, necessary to begin monitoring a designated population of children using the ASQ system. Although the figure shows a linear, one-step-at-a-time approach to planning, it is possible to work on more than one step simultaneously or to change the order of the steps.

Establish Goals and Objectives

Before a screening and monitoring program is begun, thought should be given to the goals and objectives to be accomplished. Careful delineation of the program's goals and objectives by the major stakeholders (i.e., program staff, cooperating professionals, parents, and community agencies) will help to ensure

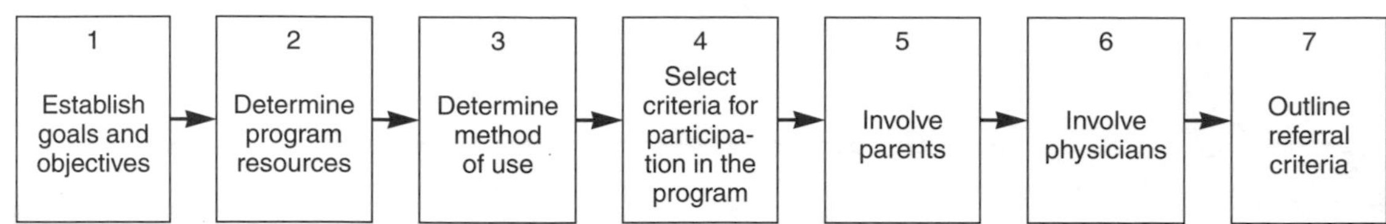

Figure 3. The planning phase of the ASQ system includes seven important steps. These steps can be performed one at a time, or a few may be undertaken simultaneously. Sometimes program staff will choose to complete the steps in an order different from the one shown here.

that the program is initiated efficiently and that day-to-day operations are effective. In addition, establishment of goals should assist in using often limited resources in the most cost-effective way. Several meetings of the participating professionals may be required to hammer out a set of reasonable and generally acceptable goals. As the amount of productive time spent during this step increases, so too does the likelihood that the program will operate satisfactorily for all involved. Although reasonable variation will occur across geographic sites, agencies, and personnel, the following goals are offered as guidelines. All, some, or none of these goals may be appropriate for particular programs.

- Early and accurate identification of infants and young children who require further evaluation
- Collaboration of community agencies to develop an effective monitoring system for children considered at risk for developmental delays or disabilities
- Increased involvement of parents in the assessment of their child's developmental progress
- Use of public health personnel to monitor the development of infants and young children considered at high risk for developmental delays or disabilities
- Community-based screening of infants and young children at designated intervals

After the program's goals have been developed, the next step is to determine the resources available to operate the program and to allocate these resources appropriately.

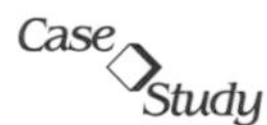

Steps-Ahead of Eugene, Oregon, is funded to provide developmental screening and monitoring of children who are at risk for developmental delays. Steps-Ahead was created to deliver screening and monitoring services to all children in Lane County. Steps-Ahead has links with other agencies in the county serving young children and their families; these links include Early Intervention Program of Lane County; Lane County Mental Health; Special Supplemental Nutrition Program for Women, Infants and Children; Kids-Kan Head Start; Child Care Resource and Referral; Butler House Alcohol and Drug Treatment Program; White Bird Homeless Shelter; Sacred Mary Hospital Newborn Intensive Care Unit; and a number of community pediatricians. Representatives from these agencies serve on an advisory board that provides ongoing advice and direction.

The primary goal of Steps-Ahead is to identify, screen, and monitor the development of all infants and children in Lane County who meet specified risk criteria. Screening and monitoring are accomplished by having parents complete the *Ages & Stages Questionnaire* for each age interval. Children are identified at 4 months and followed until their fifth birthday. Children are referred for further evaluation if their performance on the ASQ indicates a possible developmental delay. Staff identified the following objectives for Steps-Ahead's use of the ASQ system:

1. Educate referral sources about Steps-Ahead.
2. Identify, screen, and monitor referred children.
3. Educate participating families about the services of Steps-Ahead.
4. Refer children identified as having suspected delays to evaluation sources.
5. Provide Child Find and public awareness information to the community.
6. Evaluate the efforts of Steps-Ahead.

Determine Program Resources

The success of any monitoring program, no matter how low its costs, is dependent on matching its goals to available resources. Some might argue that establishing goals and determining program resources are steps best done simultaneously. If these steps are done separately, it may be necessary to revise the goals and objectives once resources are analyzed and allocated.

Determining resources may require some modification of the chosen goals and objectives in at least three ways. First, limited resources may require changes in program goals and objectives. For example, a program may have set a goal to monitor all infants discharged from the local hospital newborn intensive care unit for a period of 3 years. An examination of resources may indicate that the necessary personnel and funds are not available to conduct such a large project; however, support may be available to monitor a small subgroup of infants at extremely high risk for developmental delays (e.g., babies weighing less than 1,000 grams at birth).

Second, limited resources may require changes in the means by which a goal is accomplished. Monitoring a group of infants at risk may not be possible by conducting costly team evaluations, but it may be possible by using parents to follow their infants' development.

Third, modification of goals may be necessary when a specific resource is unavailable. For example, the goal may have been for public health nurses to assess the development of a group of infants living in low-income housing. Upon learning that the area's public health nurses are unable to take on such a responsibility, the goal must be modified by shifting the assessment activities to personnel who can take on the task.

As soon as goals are established and necessary resources are identified to meet those goals, program personnel can begin to address the specific activities needed to start a screening and monitoring program using the ASQ system.

Case Study

Steps-Ahead has one primary goal: to identify, screen, and monitor all of Lane County's children who have at least one risk factor for developmental problems. Risk factors were identified by the staff and advisory board at the inception of Steps-Ahead. Because the goals and objectives of Steps-Ahead are fairly broad, it was crucial that program resources be determined to see whether these goals could be met. The first step was to assess program resources, including personnel. The program was funded for one full-time program administrator, one full-time social worker, one half-time social worker, and one full-time secretary. Other resources, including supplies, equipment, and office space, were assessed and found to be adequate. The resources provided by the advisory board were then assessed and included the following: follow-up evaluations, professional consultation when needed, fund raising, and other in-kind support.

The next step was to evaluate these resources in terms of meeting program goals and objectives. When program staff considered the number of births in the county and the predicted percentage of participants in the program, they decided that some modification of objectives was necessary. After several meetings of the Steps-Ahead staff and the advisory board, the program's goals and objectives were amended to reflect the availability of resources. Participation was limited to families with children who were at *greatest* risk for developmental delays.

Determine Method of Use

Program staff have a number of options when deciding how to use the ASQ system. Table 1 is a compilation of strategies for using the *Ages & Stages Questionnaires.* Described next are the various ways the questionnaires can be used as part of a screening and monitoring system. The following three factors are likely to affect the method chosen:

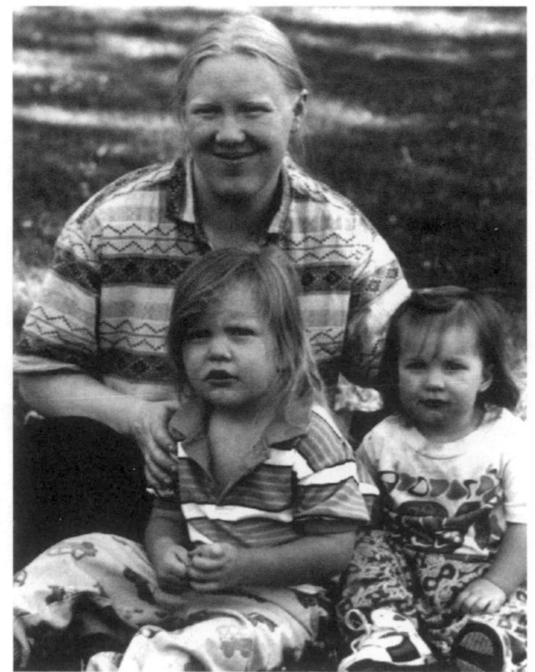

1. Type of program (e.g., state, Child Find, hospital screening, community-based early intervention)
2. Available resources (e.g., state or federal grant, assigned professional personnel, clerical support)
3. Characteristics of parents (e.g., low income, culturally diverse)

Table 1. Strategies for using the *Ages & Stages Questionnaires*

Strategy	Target population	How parent receives	Parent returns	How scored	Feedback to parents	Comments
Health and primary care setting	All children	Provided in waiting rooms or mailed 2 weeks prior to visit	On site or parent brings to exam	Nurse or clinic staff	During visit Serves as basis for discussing concerns during exam	• Need toys or materials available in waiting room • May be difficult for busy practice to mail in advance • Some families may need assistance • Language translation and cultural adaptations may be necessary • Need time to develop efficient management system by nurse or clerical staff • High involvement of primary care practitioner with system
Mail out	At risk	Mailed 1–2 weeks before "target" date of questionnaire	By mail with self-addressed, stamped envelope provided	By agency	Questionnaires that indicate suspected delay: telephone or direct contact with parents Questionnaires that do not indicate suspected delay: letter with activities for next developmental period	• May discriminate against poor readers, families from different cultural and linguistic backgrounds • May be difficult for some families at high risk • Useful in rural and remote areas
Home visit	At risk	Provided by home visitor	Completed in home	Home visitor scores with parent Summary may go to agency	During visit	• Can be used as part of home visiting curriculum • Recommended model for families at high risk and some culturally and linguistically diverse families • Toy kits available may be helpful for some families completing questionnaires

(continued)

Table 1. *(continued)*

Strategy	Target population	How parent receives	Parent returns	How scored	Feedback to parents	Comments
On site 1) Parent completes	At risk	On site • Health clinic • Child care setting • Preschool • Parenting program • Treatment center • Homeless shelter • Women, Infants, and Children (WIC)	On site	On site by service provider or with parent	On site	• Noise and on-site activity may be distracting for parents • Need toys and materials available • Parents may need assistance • Educational potential for parents and staff
2) Service provider completes or assists parents	At risk	On site • Child care setting • Preschool setting/ Head Start • Health clinic	On site or by mail	On site by service provider or with parent, if possible	On site, by telephone, or through mail	• May increase service provider's awareness of child development • Useful for "hard-to-reach" parents • Bridges communication about development • Maximizes parent involvement when completing questionnaire
Combination mail out and on site	At risk	Mailed by agency or health clinic visit	Parent brings to health clinic visit or returns by mail	By agency or staff at clinic	During visit if possible Agency can mail or telephone	• Initial face-to-face introduction of questionnaire to parents may increase accuracy and return rates • Primary care providers may be able to incorporate this screening strategy into busy office practices • Encourages medical–home connection • Requires communication and data sharing between agency and primary care provider
Combination of strategies	High risk	Parent can choose how to receive: • Home visit • Mail • Telephone • In clinic (on site) Flexibility in changing strategies, depending on family situation at the time	Choose strategy that will work for family: • On site • Home visit • Mail	By service provider or with parent, if possible	Choose strategy that will work for family: • On site • Home visit • Mail	• Personal contact and rapport may increase level of trust and cooperation • Flexibility and creativity in administration may increase reliability • Parents may require a higher level of assistance • Rewards may increase level of participation • Requires high level of involvement by service provider

A general description of each method is given here; more detailed information about each implementation method is provided in Chapter 5.

Mailing the Questionnaires Mailing the questionnaires to parents who have agreed to participate in the program is a low-cost approach for the dynamic monitoring of selected populations of infants and children at risk for developmental delays. In fact, the ASQ system was originally designed to mail out the simple-to-complete questionnaires at the preestablished intervals to parents of targeted children. Parents complete the questionnaire and mail it back to a central site for scoring by program staff.

In comparison to approaches that employ several highly skilled professionals, the cost of using the mail-out questionnaire system is extremely modest. In 1998, the Follow Along Program in Southwest Minnesota found the cost of the ASQ was $36.67 per year to mail two to three questionnaires to parents (Chan & Taylor, 1998). When indirect costs such as rent, utilities, computer hardware, and telephone fees were added, the cost per child rose to $45.80 per year. In contrast, Chan and Taylor (1998) calculated the average home visit cost by nursing staff at $78 per child. Although the materials cost is likely to be predictable across sites, regions, and states, personnel costs may vary depending on the professional level of the person mailing out and scoring the questionnaires.

One-Time Screening The ASQ system also can be used for one-time screening. Agencies with limited personnel and resources may not be able to mount a full-time monitoring program but may need to screen referred children at specific times. Although the ASQ system was developed to monitor children's development over time, the questionnaires can be used for one-time screening if resources are extremely limited.

It is preferable, however, that programs attempt ongoing monitoring of children rather than one-time screening. Other situations in which a one-time screening approach is necessary occur with programs that serve large homeless populations. For example, such a program may not have an opportunity to establish the family in the tracking program and may need to obtain more immediate feedback about the child's developmental status. When using the questionnaires with this strategy, program staff should be aware of the 2-month completion time, or "window," surrounding each questionnaire age interval. Questionnaires completed outside this window require that the child's performance on the questionnaire activities be reviewed by a professional who is knowledgeable in child development.

Interviewing The ASQ system can be used to screen children through interviews. Parents can be interviewed by a professional or other staff member in the family's home, at an office or clinic, or over the telephone. Using the questionnaires as an interview tool may be appropriate for parents with limited reading skills or poor understanding of written questions as a result of language or cognitive difficulties.

Conducting Home Visits The ASQ system can be used on home visits. Public health nurses, social workers, and other home visitors may complete the questionnaires with parents. A home visit may be required when parents are unable to read or have other difficulties with independent completion of the questionnaires or if they are unwilling to complete the questionnaires in an environment other than their home. The questionnaires may be part of a larger curriculum that is used with parents in conjunction with an abuse and neglect prevention program. Many abuse and neglect prevention programs use the questionnaires on home visits to teach parents about child development. When the questionnaires are used on a home visit, several options are available with regard to how the questionnaires are completed. The home visitor may simply assist the parent in obtaining answers for questions, or the home visitor may be more involved in questionnaire completion. It is preferable that the home visitor help parents become more independent and confident about their ability to report on their child's developmental status. In addition, the completed questionnaire can be scored in the home, either by the parents or the home visitor. Finally, the questionnaire can be left with the parents, and the home visitor can complete an Information Summary Sheet to keep for the program's records.

Involving Primary Health Care Providers The questionnaires can be used by primary health care providers as a brief screening process before a physical examination. Health care providers may save time by using the questionnaires completed by parents before the appointment because parental concerns can be identified and provide a focus for the examination.

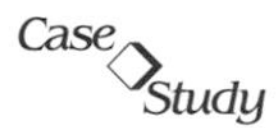

When, based on its limited resources, Steps-Ahead decided to limit participation to families at the greatest risk, staff and the advisory board needed to deviate from the usual order of the planning steps. Rather than analyzing their program resources and then determining the method of use they would follow, the Steps-Ahead staff focused on selecting participation criteria before choosing how to implement the ASQ system. Their chosen criteria are described on page 34.

When the Steps-Ahead staff returned to the decision regarding ASQ use, they carefully reviewed their options, finding it most helpful to brainstorm about how the characteristics of their families would mesh with the available resources of their program. Wanting to meet the diverse needs of families, staff opted to use a flexible approach in getting the questionnaires to parents. Mail-out, home visit, and on-site methods of administration were chosen. By allowing parents this flexibility, it was hoped that more parents would be able to participate.

Select Criteria for Participation in the Program

An important step in starting a screening and monitoring program for infants and young children is to develop objective criteria for selecting whom to monitor. Several studies have found that although biological factors play a major role in predicting severe cognitive delays, they play only a minor role in predicting mild delays. Research indicates that cumulative social and psychological factors are far more predictive of lowered intelligence and that children with multiple risk factors (e.g., teenage parents, poverty, parents with mental illness) were 24 times more likely than other children to have a lowered intelligence quotient score (Behrman, 1997; Sameroff, Seifer, Barocas, Zax, & Greenspan, 1987).

Program resources and goals must be consistent with the risk factors chosen by the screening program personnel. Programs with fewer resources may wish to target children with an increased likelihood of developmental delays. This may require selection of risk criteria that are more predictive of developmental delay. For instance, because children with more than one risk factor are more likely to need early intervention services, program personnel may focus their screening and monitoring efforts on such children. If program resources are sparse, this may be an especially compelling recommendation. Table 2 contains lists of medical and environmental/social risk criteria to aid in selecting populations considered to be at risk for developmental delays.

Table 2. Possible risk criteria for selecting populations to be monitored

Medical	Environmental/social
Gestational and perinatal	Maternal age of 19 or younger
Intracranial hemorrhage (including subdural, subarachnoid, intracerebral, intraventricular, and periventricular cystic leukomalacia)	Caregiver or infant interaction that is considered at risk
Neonatal seizures	Parents with disabilities or limited resources (including history of mental illness or disability, mental retardation, sensory impairment, incapacitating physical disability, or lack of knowledge about or ability to provide basic infant care)
Perinatal asphyxia (including one or more of the following: 5-minute Apgar score of 4 or less, no spontaneous respiration until 10 minutes of age, hypotonia persisting to 2 hours of age, and renal failure and other medical complications of asphyxia)	No or limited prenatal care
Small for gestational age (i.e., birth weight 2 standard deviations or more below the mean for gestational age)	Income below poverty level
Birth weight of 1,500 grams or less	No high school diploma
Mechanical ventilation for 72 hours or more	Atypical or recurrent accidents involving the child
Hyperbilirubinemia	Family interaction that is chronically disturbed
Central nervous system infection (including bacterial meningitis, herpes, or other viral encephalitis/meningitis)	Family with inadequate or no health care
Congenital infection (e.g., TORCH)	Lack of stable residence, homelessness, or dangerous living conditions
Congenital defect involving the central nervous system (including microcephaly, myelomeningocele)	Maternal prenatal substance abuse/use
Hydrocephalus	Parent with four or more preschool-age children
Multiple minor physical anomalies or a combination of major and minor anomalies (excluding infants with known syndromes or chromosome defects)	Parent with a developmental history of loss and/or abuse (including perinatal loss; miscarriages; sexual or physical abuse; death of parent, spouse, or child)
Abnormal neuromotor examination results at time of nursery discharge (including brachial plexus injury)	Parent with alcohol or other drug dependence
Maternal phenylketonuria or acquired immunodeficiency syndrome	Parent with severe chronic illness
Maternal alcohol or other substance abuse	Parent–child separation
Gestational age of 34 weeks or less	Physical or social isolation and/or lack of adequate social support
Aspiration pneumonia	
Family history of hearing loss	
Postnatal	
Head injury with loss of consciousness	
Central nervous system infection (including bacterial meningitis, herpes, or other viral encephalitis/meningitis)	
Nonfebrile seizures—single, prolonged, or multiple	
Failure to thrive or pediatric undernutrition (i.e., persistently slow rate of growth not associated with illness, or weight/length at the third percentile or less)	
Recurrent apnea	
Chronic illness	
Chronic otitis media (i.e., middle ear infections)	

Adapted from Benn (1993).

Other useful considerations when determining risk criteria for a screening and monitoring program include the following:

- Eligibility rules for early intervention: Under the Individuals with Disabilities Education Act Amendments of 1997 (PL 105-17), each U.S. state has identified eligibility criteria for determining developmental delays in young children. A psychometric criterion (e.g., 2 standard deviation units below the mean on a standardized measure) is often used. In addition, informed clinical opinion (e.g., a physician's statement of severe health impairment) can be the basis of eligibility determination.
- The risk criteria of other state or local screening, tracking, or monitoring programs
- Availability of resources for children identified as having developmental delays

When risk criteria are chosen, many factors must be considered. As program personnel evaluate the effectiveness of their system, it may be necessary to add or delete risk factors based on the percentages of children being identified (see Chapter 6).

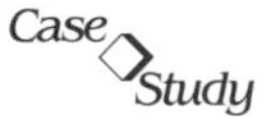

The Steps-Ahead staff acknowledged their limited resources by modifying their original goal of screening and monitoring all children with at least one risk factor. After consulting with the advisory board, Steps-Ahead staff decided they must limit the number of families they would serve. To do this, the criteria to participate in the program were changed. Instead of one risk factor, two risk factors, at least one of which was environmental, were required to qualify an infant for participation.

Given the change in risk criteria, staff recognized that fewer families in the community would be served. Steps-Ahead staff were prepared to refer families they were unable to serve to other community resources and programs.

Involve Parents and Caregivers

After the risk criteria are determined, the next step is to develop procedures for notifying parents that their infant or child is eligible to participate and to seek their active involvement in the monitoring program.

Obtaining Consent Obtaining consent from a child's parent or guardian is an important prerequisite for participation in the program. Personnel have three options for obtaining consent: 1) telephone the parent or guardian to obtain initial consent, then include a written consent form with the first questionnaire; 2) send a letter to the parent or guardian; or 3) obtain written consent in person. The way in which the initial approach to parents or guardians is made depends on the program's goals and resources. It is important to provide parents with as much information as possible about the screening and monitoring program when obtaining their consent to participate.

Figure 4 is an example of a letter that could be sent to a parent or other caregiver. It contains a brief description of the importance of early development and of the monitoring program. The letter also explains the amount of parent participation expected and the activities of the program personnel. Appendix C contains this and other letters in Spanish.

Dear [fill in parents' or guardians' names]:

The first 5 years of life are very important to your child because this time sets the stage for success in school and later life. During infancy and early childhood, many experiences should be gained and many skills learned. It is important to ensure that each child's development is proceeding without problem during this period; therefore, we are interested in helping you follow your infant's growth and development. You can help us by completing a questionnaire that will be mailed to you at 2-, 4-, or 6-month intervals. You will be asked to answer questions about some things your child can and cannot do, and to mail the questionnaire back to [fill in staff member's name].

If the completed questionnaire indicates that your baby is developing without problems, we will send a letter stating that your child's development appears typical. We will mail the next age-level questionnaire to you at the appropriate time.

If there are concerns about your baby, we will contact you directly, and you may wish to have your baby's doctor or another agency conduct a further examination. All information about your baby and your family will be kept confidential.

Sincerely,

[fill in staff member's name]
[fill in program name]

Figure 4. A sample information and agreement letter to parents or guardians. This letter should be modified by personnel to reflect the ASQ method(s) to be used by the program. A Spanish translation of this letter is provided in Appendix C.

Figure 5 is an example of a form to be completed and signed by parents or guardians indicating their willingness to participate in the screening and monitoring program. The form also gives parents and guardians the option of refusing to participate. Like Figure 4, this form should be modified as necessary to meet the specific needs of the program. It, too, is provided in Spanish in Appendix C.

Collecting Demographic Information After parents or guardians have signed a form indicating their wish to participate in the screening and monitoring program, a staff member should describe in more detail the procedures used in the program. At this time, parents should be asked to provide demographic information about their child and family. Ideally, this information is obtained in person, but it also can be gathered over the telephone or

______ I have read the description of the monitoring program, and I wish to participate. I am willing to fill out questionnaires about my child's development and mail them back promptly.

______ I have read the description of the monitoring project. I understand the purpose of this project and do not wish to participate.

Parent's or guardian's signature ____________________

Date ____________

Child's name ____________________

Child's birthdate ____________

Child's primary physician ____________________

Figure 5. A sample of a participation agreement to be signed by a child's parent or guardian before beginning implementation procedures (see Chapter 5). A Spanish translation of this form is provided in Appendix C.

Child and Family Demographic Information Sheet

1. ID # ____________________
2. Child's name ____________________
   Parent's or guardian's name (last, first) ____________________
3. Address: Number, street ____________________
   Town/city ____________________
   County ____________ State ____________ ZIP ____________
   Telephone: Home ____________
   Work ____________
4. Child's date of birth (month/day/year) _____/_____/_____
5. Child's sex (male/female) ____________
6. Child's gestational age, if known (in weeks) ____________
7. Child's birth weight (in pounds/ounces) ____________
8. Ethnicity of child ____________

---

9. In neonatal intensive care unit? (yes/no) ____________
   Length of time (in days) ____________
10. Date of admission to monitoring program (month/day/year) _____/_____/_____
11. Child status:
    At risk? (yes/no) ____________
    If yes, list three primary risk factors per category:
    Medical risk factors ____________
    Environmental risk factors ____________
    Disability?(yes/no) ____________ Disability (list) ____________
12. Is this an adoptive or foster family? (yes/no) ____________

---

13. Age of biological mother (in years) ____________
14. Mother's birth surname ____________
15. Mother's marital status ____________
16. Main wage earner ____________
17. Highest level of education of mother ____________
18. Highest level of education of partner ____________
19. Occupation of mother ____________
20. Occupation of partner ____________
21. Estimated yearly family income ____________

---

22. Physician ____________
    Telephone (or name of clinic) ____________
23. Expected due date (month/day/year) _____/_____/_____
24. Did child have any medical problems at birth? (yes/no) _____
    If yes, explain ____________
25. Has child had any medical or developmental problems since birth? (yes/no) ____________
    If yes, explain ____________
26. Total number of children in family ____________

Figure 6. A sample Child and Family Demographic Information Sheet. This form or one like it should be easily accessible throughout the child's involvement in the program. A Spanish translation of this form is provided in Appendix C.

Information Sheet. Before using this form, staff should review it carefully to make modifications necessary to meet the specific information needs of the program.

Figure 7 is a sample Child and Family Demographic Information Update Sheet. It, or a similar form, can be used to update demographic information annually or at greater or smaller intervals, depending on the program's needs.

Child and Family Demographic Information Update Sheet

1. ID # ______________
2. Child's name ______________
   Parent's or guardian's name (last, first) ______________
3. Address: Number, street ______________
   Town/city ______________
   County ______________ State ______________ ZIP ______________
   Telephone: Home ______________
   Work ______________
4. Child's date of birth (month/day/year) _____/_____/_____
5. Child's sex (male/female) ______________
6. Date of admission to monitoring program (month/day/year) _____/_____/_____
7. Parent's or guardian's marital status ______________
8. Main wage earner ______________
9. Highest level of education of mother ______________
10. Highest level of education of partner ______________
11. Occupation of mother ______________
12. Occupation of partner ______________
13. Estimated yearly family income ______________
14. Total number of children in family ______________

Figure 7. A sample Child and Family Demographic Information Update Sheet. This form or one like it should be completed as necessary throughout the child's involvement in the program. A Spanish translation of this form is provided in Appendix C.

Explaining the Screening and Monitoring Process In addition to the information provided in a letter like the one in Figure 4, program staff should provide parents with an expanded verbal or written description of the monitoring program. It is important that parents' questions and concerns be addressed. It is equally important to ensure that parents understand the program and the options available to them. Parents' willingness to be (and remain) involved in the program may hinge on understanding expectations for their involvement. Programs with extremely limited resources, which preclude personal contact, may wish to send a brief letter to parents describing the program. If the program is mailing the questionnaires, this letter may accompany the first one (ideally, 4 months). If another option is being used (e.g., home visits, one-time screening, primary health care provider monitoring), the letter may accompany an appointment card. In any case, the letter should indicate that the parent or guardian can speak to a staff member to ask specific questions.

Once parents have a general understanding of the program, the next step is to assist them in becoming familiar with the questionnaires and the specific procedures used to complete them. The following points should be included when discussing the questionnaires with parents:

1. Explain that the questionnaires are designed to determine what their child can and cannot do. Be sure they understand that their child may not be able to do all of the activities targeted in the questionnaire items.
2. Emphasize the importance of trying each activity with their child.

2. Emphasize the importance of trying each activity with their child.
3. Explain that each question in the first five sections has three possible responses, which should be checked as appropriate (see Figure 8):
   - *Yes,* meaning the child is doing the activity now
   - *Sometimes,* meaning the child is just beginning to do the activity
   - *Not yet,* meaning the child has not started to do the activity

   The Overall section contains questions to be answered by checking *yes* or *no,* and if indicated, by explaining the response.
4. Clarify how to answer questions about activities the child did earlier but no longer does or does infrequently. For example, the item may ask about crawling, but the baby now walks instead of crawls; or the baby may sit independently, but the item may ask about leaning on the hands for support while sitting. In situations like these, parents should answer *yes.* (Some parents may forget or not understand this aspect of responding; scoring will need to be modified by program personnel when this occurs, as explained in Chapter 5.)
5. Stress the importance of completing the questionnaires on time. This is more relevant for parents who will be filling out the questionnaires at home and returning them to the program by mail. Be sure that parents know whom to contact if they have questions or concerns. Each questionnaire has a space to indicate the name, address, and telephone number of the program and the name of a contact person employed by the program.

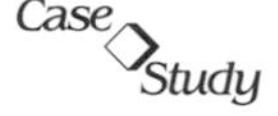

The Steps-Ahead staff decided their initial contact with parents would be within 1 month of the baby's birth. Based on information on the birth certificate completed in the hospital, the social worker determined whether the family met the required risk criteria. The social worker then sent a letter to the parents that explained the program. Within 1 week, she telephoned the parents to answer any questions they might have and to schedule a home visit. During the home visit, the Steps-Ahead social worker obtained the parents' consent to participate, enrolled the family, and described how to complete the questionnaires. The social worker also had parents choose whether they wanted to receive the questionnaires during home visits, on site, or by mail.

YES	SOMETIMES	NOT YET	
❑	❑	❑	___
❑	❑	❑	___

Figure 8. For the five areas of development (communication, gross motor, fine motor, problem solving, and personal-social), each question should be answered by checking *yes, sometimes,* or *not yet,* as shown in the columns here.

Involve Physicians

Physicians in most communities wish to be kept informed about their young patients' participation in screening and monitoring programs. Physicians may provide a developmental assessment of their patients if required or may want to be notified if an assessment is conducted by another community agency. Figure 9 is a sample letter to a physician from a program staff member, explaining the family's participation in the monitoring program.

In most cases, the staff of screening and monitoring programs will find it useful to involve physicians of participating children for two important reasons. First, physicians have valuable information about their patients, and young children in general, that may serve to enhance monitoring efforts. Second, collaboration among professionals and program personnel will produce the greatest benefits for young children and their families.

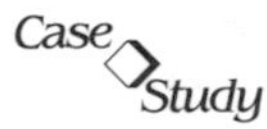

Steps-Ahead involved physicians both as participants on the advisory board and with individual families when needed. The two physicians serving on the advisory board wrote letters to other physicians in the community describing the Steps-Ahead program. To ensure physician participation, Steps-Ahead staff notified physicians when families who were the physicians' patients enrolled in the program. (Parents indicate their child's physician on the ASQ Child and Family Demographic Information Sheet.) Steps-Ahead staff also notified physicians of developmental concerns for their patients when such results were indicated by the questionnaires.

Outline Referral Criteria

The *Ages & Stages Questionnaires* are useful only if they generally identify children who require further evaluation (i.e., children who score below a cutoff point) and generally exclude children who do not (i.e., children who score at or above a cutoff point). The purpose of scoring the questionnaires is to determine which children need further assessment and which do not. The cutoff points

Dear Dr. [fill in physician's name]:

The parents or guardian of your patient [fill in child's name] have agreed to participate in a developmental monitoring program. The purpose of this project is to provide follow-along screening to infants and children who are at risk for developmental delays. Parents or guardians are asked to respond to questions about their child's development at repeated intervals from 4 months to 5 years. They answer items about activities their child can and cannot yet do. If a child obtains a score below the established cutoff on a questionnaire, the parent, or guardian, and physician are notified so that further evaluation can be scheduled.

If you would like more information about the project, please contact [fill in staff member's name].

Sincerely,

[fill in staff member's name]
[fill in program name]

Figure 9. A sample letter to a physician from a program staff member.

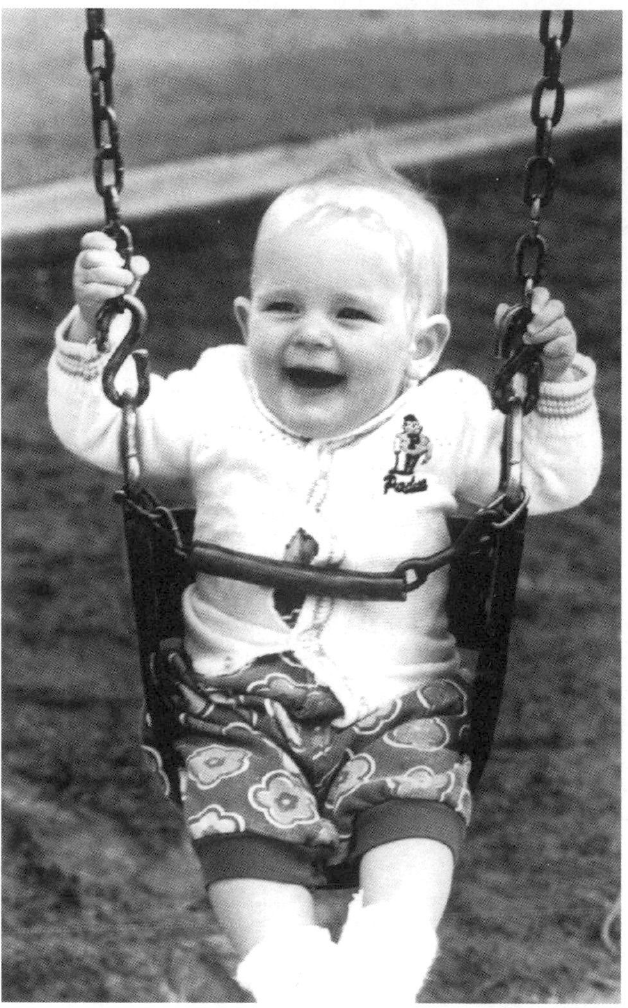

used to score the questionnaires (see Chapter 5) are markers that separate children who require referral and assessment from those who do not.

A standard cutoff point, or referral criterion, for each questionnaire age interval and for the five areas of development has been determined statistically using data from approximately 7,900 questionnaires. Using these data, the mean and standard deviation for each area of development were calculated and are contained in Table 3. The cutoff points discussed in Chapter 5 were derived by subtracting 2 standard deviations from the mean for each area of development on each questionnaire. This number was then multiplied by 10 to simplify the scoring of the questionnaires by eliminating calculations using a decimal point.

A variety of best-fit measures (i.e., relative or receiver operating characteristic [ROC] analyses, which are discussed further in Appendix F) were employed to obtain the ideal balance between overreferral and underreferral. To accomplish this, different cutoff points were tried until sensitivity and specificity were maximized. Using cutoff points of 2 standard deviations below the mean[1] was found to produce the best balance between overreferral and underreferral. (A detailed discussion of how cutoff points were established is contained in Appendix F.) The recommended referral criteria outlined next are based on this balance.

- *Refer* a child whose score in one or more areas is below the established cutoff point (i.e., 2 standard deviations below the mean) for that questionnaire interval.
- *Follow up* with a child whose score in a particular area is close to the cutoff point.
- *Follow up* with a child whose scores are above the cutoff points for each area but whose parent has indicated a concern in the Overall section of the questionnaire.

After a child's areas scores have been calculated for a specific questionnaire, they can be compared with the established cutoff points. (A table listing the cutoff points for each questionnaire is provided in Chapter 5.)

[1]The communication areas on the 14, 16, 18, 20, 22, 24, 27, 30, and 33 month questionnaires were initially excepted from this rule. For these, one additional item (10 points) was added to the cutoff scores. (However, cutoff scores for certain intervals were updated in 2004, and the new communication area cutoffs for 27 and 33 months were derived by subtracting 2 standard deviations from the mean. The new cutoffs are shown in Table 3.)

Table 3. Means and standard deviations by questionnaire for each developmental area

Age interval (months)[a]	*N*	Area	Mean	Standard deviation
4	1,380	Communication	50.7	8.7
	1,380	Gross motor	55.3	7.6
	1,380	Fine motor	43.9	10.9
	1,380	Problem solving	53.4	9.2
	1,380	Personal-social	51.2	9.1
8	1,285	Communication	53.5	8.4
	1,285	Gross motor	50.5	13.1
	1,285	Fine motor	54.4	8.8
	1,285	Problem solving	51.7	9.7
	1,285	Personal-social	51.3	10.4
12	1,091	Communication	42.2	13.2
	1,091	Gross motor	48.6	15.3
	1,091	Fine motor	49.2	10.4
	1,091	Problem solving	48.6	11.7
	1,091	Personal-social	45.5	12.7
16	976	Communication	49.1	12.3
	976	Gross motor	55.3	11.5
	976	Fine motor	51.8	10.6
	976	Problem solving	49.7	11.4
	976	Personal-social	48.5	10.9
20	845	Communication	47.7	10.7
	845	Gross motor	55.4	9.6
	845	Fine motor	54.4	7.3
	845	Problem solving	49.1	9.6
	845	Personal-social	52.8	8.8
24	820	Communication	49.5	11.5
	820	Gross motor	54.4	9.2
	820	Fine motor	52.8	8.2
	820	Problem solving	51.5	9.3
	820	Personal-social	52.4	8.4
30	562	Communication	55.8	8.5
	562	Gross motor	51.2	10.3
	562	Fine motor	49.8	12.3
	562	Problem solving	50.9	11.0
	562	Personal-social	52.7	7.9
36	512	Communication	54.3	7.8
	512	Gross motor	54.7	9.5
	512	Fine motor	52.5	10.9
	512	Problem solving	55.0	8.2
	512	Personal-social	53.5	7.4
48[b]	336	Communication	55.9	8.4
	336	Gross motor	52.5	9.5
	336	Fine motor	43.5	14.3
	336	Problem solving	56.7	8.1
	336	Personal-social	48.6	12.6
60	125	Communication	49.9	9.1
	125	Gross motor	52.3	9.8
	125	Fine motor	51.1	10.3
	125	Problem solving	51.3	10.6
	125	Personal-social	54.1	7.3

Note: This table was updated in 2005. The data reported in previous printings of this table may vary slightly from the data in this table due to rounding errors.

[a]The optional questionnaires (6, 10, 14, 18, 22, 27, 33, 42, and 54 months) were not included in this analysis.

[b]On the 48 month ASQ, the cutoff scores for fine motor and problem solving were adjusted using a statistical technique called the receiver operating characteristic, discussed further in Appendix F.

Although the cutoff points presented in Chapter 5 were empirically derived using a large number of questionnaires, it is important to emphasize that programs may have legitimate reasons to determine their own screening criteria and to adjust the empirically derived cutoff points. Furthermore, it should be stressed that there are no cutoff scores (or screening tests) that will not result in errors of underreferral and overreferral. The empirically derived cutoff points shown in Chapter 5 were chosen to minimize underreferral and overreferral; however, these cutoff points may not be ideal for all monitoring programs. Program staff should adjust their referral criteria or cutoff points so that children who are identified as having problems do, in fact, require further evaluation.

There are at least two categories of factors that may require modification of a program's referral criteria:

1. Risk factors associated with the populations to be monitored
2. Resources available to the program

Program personnel may wish to adjust their cutoff points if they are tracking a group of children who are at extreme risk (e.g., birth weight less than 1,000 grams) or who have multiple risk factors (e.g., low birth weight, teenage parents, low income). Adjustments may also be in order if programs have few resources (e.g., only a part-time staff member to score questionnaires and make follow-up telephone calls) or if programs have extensive resources (e.g., several personnel available to make follow-up telephone calls and home visits). Finally, adjustments may be necessary if there are limited evaluation resources and/or eligibility criteria for services are extremely high (e.g., only one evaluation center, which has long waiting lists; services limited to children with severe disabilities).

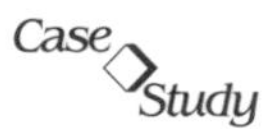

Steps-Ahead decided to use the referral criteria in *The ASQ User's Guide.* Children with one or more areas below the cutoff point were referred to the Early Intervention Program of Lane County for a developmental evaluation. If these children did not qualify for the early intervention program, then Steps-Ahead continued to monitor them using the ASQ system. When a child's score was close to the cutoff point in any area on the questionnaires, parents were given ideas for games that would help build the child's skills in that area. The child's development continued to be monitored by Steps-Ahead. When a child had one or more questionnaires with parent concerns marked in the Overall section, the social worker contacted the parent and discussed the concerns. Based on the discussion, the child continued to be monitored by Steps-Ahead or was referred for developmental evaluation, or the family was linked with other needed services.

CONCLUSION

As previously mentioned, time devoted to the planning steps described in this chapter is well spent in terms of ensuring the long-term success of a screening and monitoring program. The seven steps in this phase provide a foundation on which the day-to-day activities of using the ASQ system with young children and with families can take place. In the next chapter, these daily activities are described in detail. Assembling child files, using a tickler system, scoring questionnaires, and determining follow-up criteria are among the activities described. Forms to assist with organizing and maintaining the monitoring system are included.

5

Phase II: Using and Scoring the Questionnaires

ASQ™

After the planning phase of the ASQ process is completed, program personnel can move into Phase II, the implementation of screening and monitoring procedures. This phase, primarily focused on using and scoring the questionnaires, has five important steps. Figure 10 provides an overview of the steps in Phase II, and this chapter defines each step and describes its component parts.

STEPS IN PHASE II: USING AND SCORING THE QUESTIONNAIRES

Assemble the Child File

Assembling individual files for each participant ensures that all questionnaires and forms concerning the family and the child's progress will be kept in a single location so, when necessary, information can be obtained efficiently. For example, forms containing child and family demographic information (e.g., a form similar to the one shown in Figure 6 on p. 36) should be kept in the front of the file because they may be needed frequently. All of the information in the file should be updated periodically using a form like the one shown in Figure 7 on page 37.

Developing a child file is best accomplished by completing the following steps:

1. Assign the child an identification (ID) number. The first child to join the program might be assigned the number 001, the second 002, and so forth. ID numbers should be assigned for two reasons. First, children with the same or similar last names are less likely to be confused if ID numbers are assigned. Second, the use of ID numbers can ensure confidentiality when necessary.
2. Place the Child and Family Demographic Information Sheet at the front of the file. If, for some reason, these data have not been collected yet, they should be obtained before proceeding.
3. Complete a Child Information Summary Sheet, on which are recorded basic identifying data (see Figure 11). Add this form to the child file.
4. If the child was born more than 3 weeks prematurely, calculate his or her corrected date of birth. The corrected date of birth should be used until the child's chronological age is 24 months. Record the corrected date of

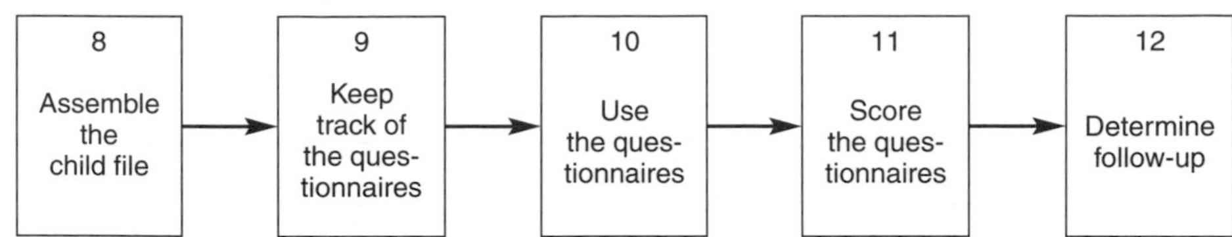

Figure 10. The second phase of the ASQ system contains five steps. While focusing on this implementation phase, staff are screening and monitoring participating children for developmental delays and are making recommendations for referral when indicated by questionnaire scores.

birth on the Child Information Summary Sheet. A child's corrected date of birth (CDOB) is calculated by adding the weeks of prematurity to the child's date of birth.

5. Enter the child's name and ID number on the program's Master List Form. Figure 12 is a blank Master List Form that may be photocopied and modified to meet the needs of specific programs. This list of participating children is essential to the smooth and efficient operation of a screening and monitoring system because it assists program personnel in ensuring that necessary information is collected and questionnaires are completed.
6. Label the file with the child's name, ID number, and other information that program personnel may find essential (e.g., date of birth).
7. Store the file in an accessible but secure location.

Keep Track of the Questionnaires

When tracking large numbers of children over time, it is essential that accurate and efficient procedures are adopted to permit timely distribution and

ID # ___________

Child Information Summary Sheet

1. Name ______________________________
2. Date of birth (month/day/year) ______/______/______
3. Sex (male/female) ______________
4. Gestational age (best estimate in weeks) ______________
5. Corrected date of birth (if applicable) ______________
6. Mother's name ______________________________
7. Partner's name ______________________________
8. Other caregiver(s) ______________________________
3. Address: Number, street ______________________________
   Town/city ______________________________
   County ______________ State ______________ ZIP __________
   Telephone: Home ______________
   Work ______________
10. Pediatrician ______________________________
11. Notes/comments ______________________________

Figure 11. The Child Information Summary Sheet should be completed during the first step of the implementation phase. It should be kept in the child's file. A Spanish translation of this form is provided in Appendix C.

Master List Form

Site ______________________________

Child name	ID#	Parent consent	Child & Family Demographic Info. Sheet	Physician info. letter	Child & Family Demographic Info. Update Sheet	Child file card	4 month ASQ	6 month ASQ	8 month ASQ	10 month ASQ	12 month ASQ	14 month ASQ	16 month ASQ	18 month ASQ	20 month ASQ	22 month ASQ	24 month ASQ	27 month ASQ	30 month ASQ	33 month ASQ	36 month ASQ	42 month ASQ	48 month ASQ	54 month ASQ	60 month ASQ

Figure 12. Program staff should be diligent in keeping the Master List Form up-to-date. Every child who is participating in the program should be listed by name and ID number on this form or one like it.

completion of questionnaires. The integrity of the ASQ system is dependent on reasonable adherence to a preset schedule. The schedule ensures that the parent or service provider who will complete the questionnaire receives it 1 or 2 weeks before the child reaches the indicated age interval to be tested (i.e., 4, 6, 8, 10, 12, 14, 16, 18, 20, 22, 24, 27, 30, 33, 36, 42, 48, 54, and 60 months). For infants born prematurely, the corrected age should be used when completing the questionnaires until the baby is 24 months old.

The method of use selected by the program or agency (see Chapter 4) will affect the way in which questionnaires are distributed and used; however, some general guidelines do apply to all uses. First, the program or agency name, address, and telephone number should be typed or stamped on the first page of the questionnaire before it is mailed. Space is provided in the middle of this page where the image of the mother and child appears. (Figure 13 presents an example for Steps-Ahead, the program featured in the case study in Chapter 4.) Once the monitoring system is operational, staff may wish to enter this information on all of the master questionnaires upon receipt. This strategy is likely to work, although staff should realize that this information may need to be updated if any of the program's identifying information should change.

Second, timely questionnaire distribution and receipt can be accomplished through use of a card file tickler system that is adaptable to a mail-back system and other uses of the questionnaires. The following directions provide general instructions on the use of such a system for mailing questionnaires.

Card File Tickler System To begin, locate a 5" x 8" index card (or other size) file box. Place dividers for each month (e.g., January, February, March), with weekly subdividers included for each month, in the file box. Programs may choose to arrange the subdividers by day, week, biweekly interval, or month, depending on the number of children monitored. Complete an individual index card for each child monitored in the program. Figure 14 shows a sample card for a child named Joseph Henry; a blank sample card is provided as well for program staff to photocopy on an as-needed basis. The card contains space to record essential identifying information for the child and family, as well as a tracking grid to assist program staff.

The sample grid includes a column listing the program's planned activities in the order they are to be administered and columns for each age interval at which a questionnaire is to be completed. Upon completion of each activity in the first column, staff enter the date in the appropriate column. The

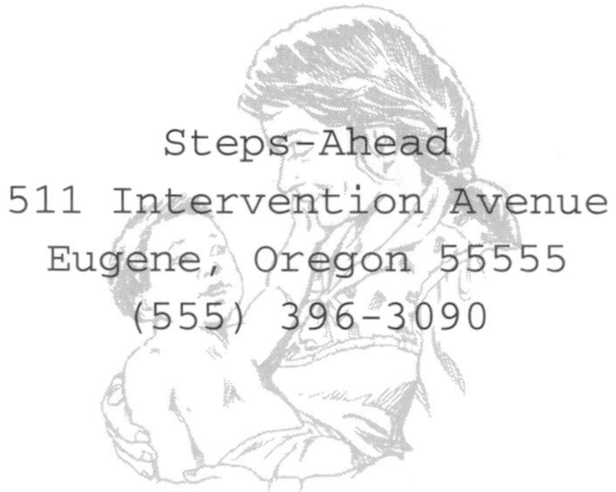

Figure 13. On the first page of each questionnaire, important program identifying information should be added. In this example, the staff at Steps-Ahead have entered the program's name, address, and telephone number for the easy reference of parents and service providers.

Child's name Joseph Henry

Parent's or guardian's name Pam & Gerald Henry

Address 22 Lakeside, Cottage Grove, OR 97461

Telephone 235-9166 Message None

Corrected date of birth None

Child's sex M

Date of birth Sept. 22, 1998

ACTIVITIES	4 MO	6 MO	8 MO	10 MO	12 MO	14 MO	16 MO	18 MO	20 MO	22 MO	24 MO	27 MO	30 MO	33 MO	36 MO	42 MO	48 MO	54 MO	60 MO
Send questionnaire					9-15-99		1-15-00												
Sent questionnaire					9-15-99														
Call—instructions					9-19-99														
Called					9-19-99														
Expected return					9-22-99														
Returned					9-25-99														
If not, called																			
Results					OK														
Feedback sent					9-28-99														
Parent called with concern					—														
Physician notified					—														
Referral					—														
Refile card (y/n)					Y														

Comments:

(continued)

Figure 14. The card file tickler system includes a card for each child participating in the program. As shown on this sample card completed for Joseph Henry, essential identifying information is recorded, and staff use the grid to track the distribution and return of questionnaires. Basic results are also recorded. The blank card on the next page may be photocopied for program use.

Figure 14. *(continued)*

Child's name ______ Corrected date of birth ______
Parent's or guardian's name ______ Child's sex ______
Address ______ Date of birth ______
Telephone ______ Message ______

ACTIVITIES	4 MO	6 MO	8 MO	10 MO	12 MO	14 MO	16 MO	18 MO	20 MO	22 MO	24 MO	27 MO	30 MO	33 MO	36 MO	42 MO	48 MO	54 MO	60 MO
Send questionnaire																			
Sent questionnaire																			
Call—instructions																			
Called																			
Expected return																			
Returned																			
If not, called																			
Results																			
Feedback sent																			
Parent called with concern																			
Physician notified																			
Referral																			
Refile card (y/n)																			

Comments:

activities column contains entries for follow-up, which may not be necessary if the questionnaire is completed and returned to the program on schedule. After a questionnaire is mailed or given to the parents, the card is refiled in chronological order under the month and week the questionnaire should be returned. All activities associated with tracking the child's progress are filed by date under the appropriate month and week.

For example, Joseph's card, which is shown in Figure 14, is filed under the week of September 15 because that date is 1 week before Joseph will become 12 months old. When September 15 arrives, the card is reviewed, and Joseph's parents are sent a 12 month questionnaire. A notation is made on the card indicating that a reminder call should be made to the parents on September 19, approximately 4–5 days after the questionnaire was mailed, and that the questionnaire should be returned by September 22. The card is filed under the week of September 19 until the call is made and the questionnaire is returned.

If the questionnaire arrives before September 22, this is indicated on the card. In addition, other important information should be recorded on the card when possible (e.g., feedback sent, results of questionnaire, whether child was referred for services). A space is also provided at the bottom of the card to record any additional comments or information relevant to the child. The date for mailing the next questionnaire is recorded, and the card is refiled under the appropriate month and day.

Joseph's parents returned the questionnaire on September 25; the results indicated typical development, and staff sent feedback to them on September 28. Joseph's parents are scheduled to receive a 16 month questionnaire next, thus the card is refiled under the week of January 15, approximately 4 months after the last questionnaire was completed. If Joseph's parents had not returned the questionnaire by September 29, they would have been called, and a new expected return date would have been recorded with the card being filed under this new date.

Specific steps for following this system are outlined next. In all steps, "target" refers to the assigned date for completing the questionnaire; for premature infants under 24 months of age, this number reflects the corrected age rather than the chronological date of birth.

1. Enter child's name and additional identifying information at the top of the card. If the child was premature, be sure to verify the CDOB before completing this entry.
2. Enter the target date minus 1–2 weeks under the appropriate age interval column to indicate when the questionnaire should be mailed or given to the parents or service providers who will be completing the form. File the card in the box under that date.
3. Mail or give the questionnaire to the parents or service provider 1–2 weeks before the target date. Record the date the questionnaire is mailed or given to whomever will be completing it.
4. If program resources permit, plan to call the parents or service providers completing the questionnaire 1 or 2 days before the target date. File the card under the date when this call should be made. During this telephone call, answer any questions and encourage prompt return of the questionnaire. Record the date of this conversation on the child's file card. Calculate the expected date of return, which is the target date plus 1–2 weeks, and enter this date on the card. Refile the child's card under the target date.

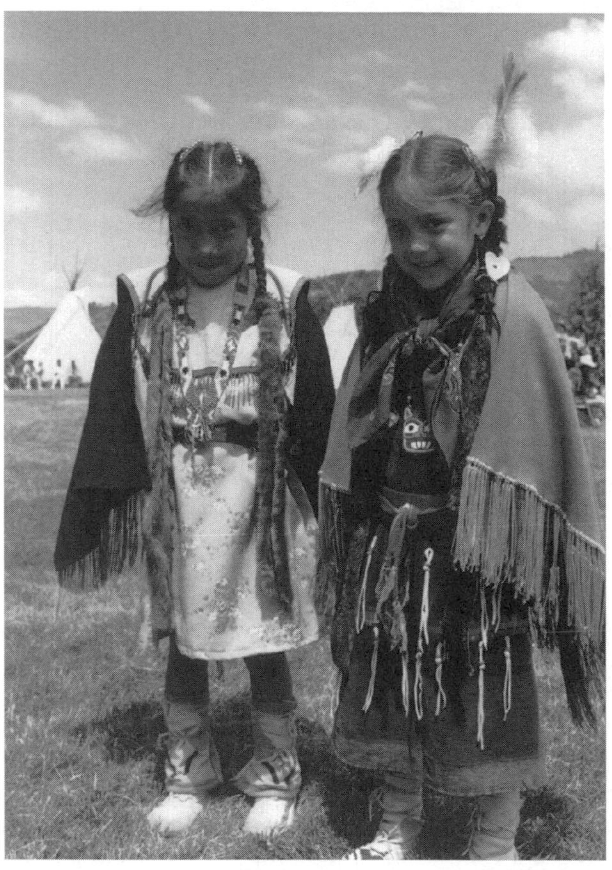

5. If the questionnaire is returned on or before the expected return date, record the date it is received.
6. If the questionnaire has not been returned by the expected return date, call the parents or service provider who agreed to complete the questionnaire. If resources permit, call again 3 or 4 days later if the questionnaire still has not been returned. If the parents cannot be reached by telephone, send a reminder in the mail. If the parents cannot be contacted by any means, make a note of this and the reasons (e.g., telephone disconnected).
7. Score the questionnaire (see the instructions on pp. 66–78), and record the results on the file card (e.g., referral, ok).
8. If the questionnaire results indicated typical development (ok), provide feedback to the parents. (A prototype letter is shown in English in Figure 20 on p. 78 and in Spanish in Appendix C.) If the child's questionnaire scores meet the referral criteria determined by the program (see pp. 39–42), begin referral procedures discussed on pages 78–84.
9. If a referral is made, note the date on the child's file card and proceed according to the guidelines discussed on page 84.
10. If a referral is not made, file the card under the next target date.

For the purposes of keeping the program up to date, a Child and Family Demographic Information Update Sheet should be completed by a parent at 12, 24, 36, 48, and 54 months. The most efficient way to obtain this information may be to mail or give this update form to the parents along with the questionnaire for that age interval and to request its return with the completed questionnaire.

Use the Questionnaires

As mentioned in Chapter 2, one advantage of using the *Ages & Stages Questionnaires* to monitor child development is the system's flexibility. This section addresses specific considerations for each use of the system.

Preparation of the Questionnaires As mentioned previously and shown in Figure 13, the first page of each questionnaire provides a space for programs to stamp, type, or write essential identifying information. Some programs may choose to affix or stamp a logo as well. Identifying information is vital when mail-out procedures are used. The name of a contact person may be indicated as well to give parents access to a resource who can answer their questions or address their concerns.

The first page of each questionnaire also contains a summary of "important points to remember"; this list reminds parents to try to make questionnaire completion a game for the family to enjoy and provides a space for staff to indicate when the next questionnaire should be expected.

The second page of each questionnaire contains a list of questions for the parent to complete. In addition to identifying information about the child and family, the answers to these questions will aid staff by indicating who is filling out the questionnaire at each interval.

The next three or four pages (depending on the age interval) of the ASQ contain the questionnaire items, which, as explained in Chapter 3, are arranged from easiest to most difficult behavior in five areas: communication, gross motor, fine motor, problem solving, and personal-social. Each item is intended to be answered by checking a box in the columns labeled *yes, sometimes,* or *not yet.* A few of the items include space for the parent to write an example of the child's behavior. The final questionnaire page contains the Overall section, which contains six questions to be answered by checking *yes* or *no.* Depending on the response, an explanation may be requested.

The final page of each questionnaire is the Information Summary Sheet. This page is optional, and program staff will need to decide whether they want to include it for family members to complete. Many programs will not send this page to parents but will instead use it as a record for their files. This sheet was designed to be used in screening programs that have personal contact with parents, such as those using the interview or home visit procedures described next. The Information Summary Sheet contains identifying information about the child and family, an abbreviated Overall section, instructions for scoring the questionnaire, a bar graph indicating cutoff scores for referral, and an item-by-item grid for recording responses to the individual questions on the previous pages.

Mail-Out Procedures The ASQ system was originally developed to be used in a mail-out format. This system fits the needs of programs that screen children whose parents are capable of reading, observing and indicating their children's behaviors, and mailing back the questionnaires.

In each master set of questionnaires, a master mail-out and mail-back sheet is provided. For programs that decide to use this format, the name of the screening program and its address should be stamped, printed, or typed on the mail-back page; and the parent's name and address should be written or typed on the mail-out page (as shown in Figure 15). Once the identifying information for the child is completed and the questionnaire is ready to be mailed out, the questionnaire may be stapled or taped at the ends and top. Staff may prefer to use an envelope to mail the questionnaires; in these cases, a stamped return envelope should also be enclosed to encourage return of the completed questionnaires.

The *Ages & Stages Questionnaires* are designed to be photocopied as needed by program staff.[1] Each master questionnaire features a different color

[1]*Purchasers of the* ***Ages & Stages Questionnaires®: A Parent-Completed, Child-Monitoring System*** *are granted permission to photocopy the questionnaires as well as the sample letters and forms in* ***The ASQ User's Guide for the Ages & Stages Questionnaires®: A Parent-Completed, Child-Monitoring System*** *in the course of their agency's service provision to families.* Each branch office that will be using the ASQ system must purchase its own set of original questionnaires; master forms cannot be shared among sites. The questionnaires and samples are meant to be used to facilitate screening and monitoring and to assist in the early identification of children who may need further evaluation. Electronic reproduction of the questionnaires is prohibited, and none of the ASQ materials may be reproduced to generate revenue for any program or individual. Photocopies may only be made from an original set of color-coded master questionnaires and/or an original ***User's Guide***. Programs are prohibited from charging parents, caregivers, or other service providers who will be completing and/or scoring the questionnaires fees in excess of the exact cost to photocopy the master forms. This restriction is not meant to apply to reimbursement of usual and customary charges for developmental screening when performed with other evaluation and management services. The ASQ materials may not be used in a way contrary to the family-oriented philosophies of the ASQ developers. *Unauthorized use beyond this privilege is prosecutable under federal law.* You will see the copyright protection line at the bottom of each form.

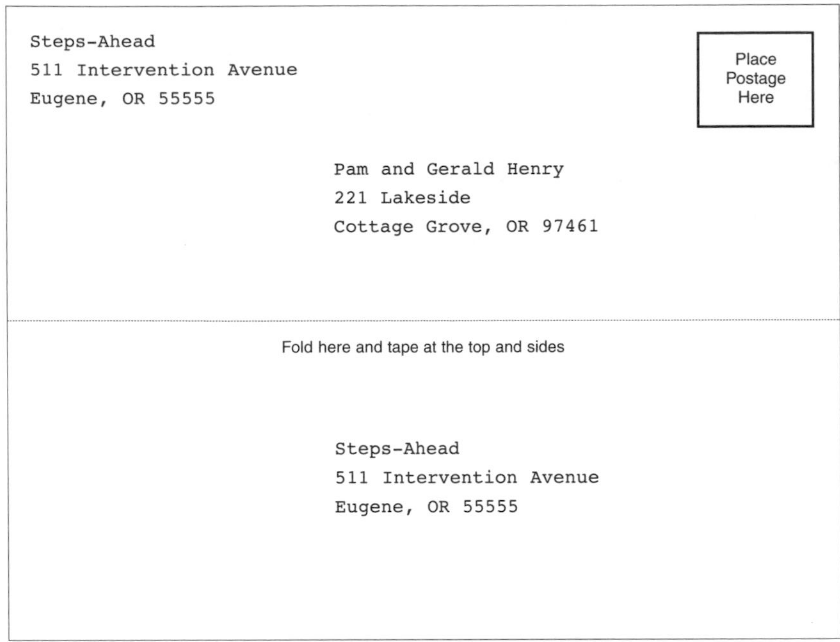
Steps-Ahead
511 Intervention Avenue
Eugene, OR 55555

Place Postage Here

Pam and Gerald Henry
221 Lakeside
Cottage Grove, OR 97461

Fold here and tape at the top and sides

Steps-Ahead
511 Intervention Avenue
Eugene, OR 55555

Figure 15. If mail-out procedures are being used, staff can use the mail-back master form provided with the *Ages & Stages Questionnaires.* The example shown here is ready to be mailed to Joseph Henry's family for questionnaire completion.

for easy visual recognition by the staff in charge of photocopying and/or distributing the questionnaires. The questionnaires may also be printed out from the *ASQ CD-ROM,* which is sold separately from the boxed questionnaires.

Return Rates A common concern in using the questionnaires in the mail-out format is their return rate. Many screening programs use the questionnaires in this format, and a variety of ideas for increasing return rates has been generated. First, it is important to follow the steps for using the tracking system described in this section. This includes making a follow-up telephone call a few days after the questionnaire is mailed to ensure receipt and to address any questions the parent might have. If a questionnaire is not returned within 2 weeks, a second telephone call should be made to remind the parent to return the questionnaire. It is equally important to adhere to the tracking schedule for sending questionnaires and feedback. Parents should be able to expect the appropriate questionnaire on time and should receive feedback in writing, by telephone, or in person within a short period. It may be important to include with the first questionnaire a welcome letter to parents, reminding them about the screening program and questionnaires.

A second option for increasing return rates is to provide incentives for parents. Incentives may be mailed to parents along with the feedback letter. For example, programs may find a local fast-food restaurant to sponsor the screening program by supplying coupons. Another idea is to include a birthday card with the questionnaires on the child's first, second, third, fourth, and fifth birthdays.

Third, staff may decide to mail an Intervention Activities Sheet, such as one of those provided in Appendix D, with the feedback letter. These sheets are designed to accompany each questionnaire and contain activities that parents may try at home. The activities sheets are also available on the *ASQ CD-ROM.*

Fourth, if resources permit, returning the questionnaires to the parents after staff have recorded scores may increase return rates by helping parents feel some "ownership" of the system. Sending the questionnaires back to parents may also increase the potential for them to learn about child development and behavior.

Specific steps designed for the use and tracking of the mail-out ASQ option are delineated next. Careful adherence to these steps is the first guideline for ensuring a high return rate:

1. Pull the child's card from the tickler file box.
2. Complete the identifying information on the first page of the questionnaire.
3. Record the questionnaire target date (i.e., the date the child will be 4 months, 8 months, etc.) under Expected Return on the tickler file card.
4. Prepare the questionnaire for mailing, either by stapling or taping the ends or by putting it in an envelope. If stapled or taped, the program's return address and a stamp should be added to the mail-back sheet. If mailed in an envelope, a program-addressed, stamped envelope should be included.
5. Record the date the questionnaire is mailed on the child's tickler file card under Sent Questionnaire.
6. Record a date 3 or 4 days after mailing in the Call—Instructions column.
7. Refile the card under the date marked in the Call—Instructions column.
8. Check the tickler file and call parents on the date marked for Call—Instructions to ensure that the questionnaire was received and to answer any questions the parents may have about completing the questionnaire.
9. Record the date the parents were contacted in the Called column.
10. Refile the tickler file card in the file box under the date in the Expected Return column.
11. If the questionnaire is returned before the expected return date, record the date returned under the column entitled Returned.
12. If the questionnaire is not returned by the expected return date, call the child's parents and record the date in the If Not, Called column.
13. Score the questionnaire according to the instructions below, and record the results on the Information Summary Sheet.
14. If the questionnaire results indicate the child is developing typically, send a feedback letter like the one in Figure 20 (or for Spanish-speaking families, a letter like the one provided in Appendix C) and an Intervention Activities Sheet from Appendix D. If program resources permit, also send parents a copy of the questionnaire.
15. If the questionnaire results indicate that a child is identified as needing an in-depth assessment, call the child's parents to discuss options.
    - Ask the parents if they want the questionnaire results sent to the child's physician.
    - When appropriate, obtain the parents' written consent to share questionnaire results with other agencies and the child's physician.
    - Refer the child for further assessment, if indicated.
    - Determine whether the child will continue to be monitored using the questionnaires. Children would be discontinued for three reasons: 1) at parent's request, 2) if the child was older than 5 years, or 3) if developmental delays were identified on the follow-up evaluation and the child was receiving early intervention services.

16. Refile the child's tickler file card under the date for the next questionnaire age interval.

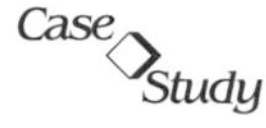

Steps-Ahead offers the mail-out procedure as an option for parents participating in the program. The Carlson family has been completing the questionnaires by mail for the last 3 years for their third child, Sarah, who was born 8 weeks early with birth complications. The Carlson family decided they would like to receive the questionnaires by mail because of their busy schedules and rural home location. Sarah's parents have completed all of the questionnaires on time, with little prompting or assistance. They receive a follow-up telephone call 3 or 4 days after each questionnaire is mailed. In the beginning, on a couple of occasions, staff reassured the Carlsons by telephone that although Sarah was not getting *yes* responses for all of the items on her questionnaires, she was still within the program's cutoff points for typical development. On Sarah's first, second, and third birthdays, Steps-Ahead sent her a birthday card as a way of recognizing Sarah and thanking the family for their participation in Steps-Ahead. Staff believe that cards and letters provide incentives for returning the next questionnaire. The Carlsons mentioned that they appreciate getting a copy of their completed ASQ with the feedback letter and that they feel reassured about Sarah's developmental progress by completing the questionnaire.

One-Time Screening Procedures Screening and monitoring programs may use the *Ages & Stages Questionnaires* as a one-time screening tool. This approach may be useful for programs with limited resources and personnel who may not be able to mount a full-time monitoring program. In addition, there may be families who are in transition and will not remain at the same address for a long enough period to enroll them in an ongoing program.

A few considerations are necessary if the questionnaires are used as a one-time screening tool. First, each questionnaire interval is valid for 1 month before and 1 month after the interval age, creating a 2-month "window" for use. For example, a 12 month questionnaire can be used between the ages of 11 and 13 months. Using the *Ages & Stages Questionnaires* with the one-time screening approach means a child may fall outside the "window" for valid scoring of the questionnaires. Although empirically derived cutoff scores are not available outside the "window," it is possible to estimate, by using clinical judgment, whether the child should be referred for further assessment. (See the discussion on Screening Children on Dates Between Questionnaire Age Intervals in this chapter for specific instructions for using the questionnaires in this manner.)

In general, a one-time screening approach will take place in the parents' home or at a clinic or office. Programs may choose to use this approach when staff believe they will not get another chance to screen a particular child. A list of materials required for use with each questionnaire can be found in Appendix E.

When staff deem it necessary to use one-time screening, the steps described here should be followed:

1. Obtain the parents' written consent to complete the questionnaire and accompanying forms.
2. Complete the Child and Family Demographic Information Sheet with the family.
3. Complete the identifying information on the second page of the questionnaire with the family.
4. Determine whether the parents are capable of reading and understanding the questionnaire.
5. If the questionnaire is to be mailed, refer to the mail-out procedures on pages 53–56.
6. If the questionnaire is to be completed on site, refer to the interviewing procedures provided in the next section.
7. If completing the questionnaires in the parents' home or living quarters, refer to the home visit procedures on pages 59–62.
8. If possible, take additional steps to arrange for further screening or assessment as needed.

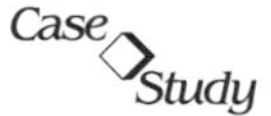

The majority of the families in the Steps-Ahead program receive questionnaires by mail or have a home visitor help to complete them. These procedures allow Steps-Ahead to track and monitor the development of children who are at risk over time. On a number of occasions, however, it has been necessary to use the questionnaires on a one-time screening basis. Carla Jones is a single mother with three children under the age of 6. At the time Carla was referred to Steps-Ahead, she was unemployed and living with her sister. Carla indicated to the staff at Steps-Ahead that she would soon be leaving the area to join her boyfriend in a county several hundred miles away. Steps-Ahead staff made a home visit and helped Carla complete the 4 month ASQ for her baby who was then 3 months old. The child's scores indicated that he was developing typically; however, staff felt that Carla was in need of additional parenting support. Carla signed a release of information form and her child's records, including the completed 4 month questionnaire, were sent to the public health program in the county to which she was moving.

Interviewing Procedures When using the questionnaires as a telephone interviewing tool, parents should have their own copy of the questionnaire. A copy of the age-appropriate questionnaire should be mailed to the parents prior to the interview so they can see the illustrations provided for some items.

The interviewer should begin by obtaining the identifying information on the second page of the questionnaire. Family information data should be updated as well, so the interviewer should have available a Child and Family Demographic Information Update Sheet. After the questions on the second page of the ASQ have been completed, the interviewer should summarize for parents the information on the first page of the questionnaire. Parents should understand that the purpose of the interview is to determine what their child can and cannot do, and that the child may not be able to do all of the activities described in the questionnaire items. The interviewer should also explain the three possible responses of *yes, sometimes,* and *not yet* for the items in the five areas of development.

When using the interview format, it is important to encourage parents to try all of the activities with their child. If a parent has difficulty answering certain items and the behavior cannot be observed at the time, the interviewer should offer to call back later after the parent has had ample time to try all of the activities.

While moving through the questionnaire items, the interviewer should identify and define each area of development (e.g., communication) and note the number of questions in each area. After completing the five sections on development, the interviewer should explain that the last section contains general, overall questions. The interviewer should remember that parents' comments are important and should be recorded.

The following steps are recommended for completing the *Ages & Stages Questionnaires* during a telephone interview:

1. Refer to the mail-out procedures on pages 53–56 for instructions to mail the questionnaire to the parents' home.
2. Call the parents 3 or 4 days after the questionnaire has been mailed.
3. Ensure that the parents have their own copy of the questionnaire as the interview is conducted.
4. Complete the Child and Family Demographic Information Sheet or Child and Family Demographic Information Update Sheet, if necessary.
5. Ask the parents for the identifying information requested on the second page of the questionnaire. The interviewer's name should be recorded along with the parents' names in response to, "Who is completing this questionnaire?"
6. Explain the purpose of the questionnaires (i.e., to determine what their child can and cannot do). Emphasize that the child is not expected to be able to do all of the activities described on the questionnaire.
7. Clarify the role of the interviewer (i.e., to read the items and describe to the parent how to observe the behavior, if necessary).
8. Explain the scoring system: *yes* indicates the child is performing the behavior; *sometimes* indicates the child is just beginning to perform the behavior (i.e., it is an emerging skill); and *not yet* indicates the child has not begun to perform the behavior.
9. While moving through the interview, introduce each area of development on the questionnaire: Communication items examine the child's language skills—both what the child understands and what the child can say; gross motor items examine large muscle movement and coordination; fine motor items examine small muscle movement and coordination; problem solving items examine the child's play with toys; and personal-social items examine the child's interaction with toys and other children.
10. Read each item on the questionnaire.
11. If the parents are unsure of how their child would perform on a particular item, offer to call back so the parents have time to try the item with

the child. Before hanging up, remind the parents of the item(s) for which a return telephone call will be made.

12. Explain and complete the Overall section of the questionnaire.
13. Using the procedures described on pages 66–78, score the questionnaire with the parents using the Information Summary Sheet or send feedback information to the parents by mail.
14. Follow the mail-out procedures on pages 53–56 for refiling the child's tickler file card.

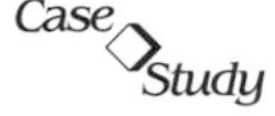

Steps-Ahead has used the interview procedure on occasion. The Briggs family lives in a very remote location, more than 2 hours by car from the Steps-Ahead office. The family indicated they prefer a home visitor, rather than receiving the questionnaire by mail; but the staff at Steps-Ahead are not able to make home visits for every questionnaire age interval. When it is not possible for a home visitor to travel to the family, the questionnaire is mailed using the mail-out procedures described previously. A social worker from Steps-Ahead then calls Mrs. Briggs and completes the questionnaire over the telephone. This approach gives the family some personal contact; and, if any questions arise, the social worker provides immediate feedback. Mrs. Briggs prefers the home visit because of the sense of isolation she experiences because of her location, but she is reassured with a telephone call from the Steps-Ahead social worker.

Home Visiting Procedures The *Ages & Stages Questionnaires* can be adapted for use on home visits. The home visitor should begin by introducing him- or herself and the monitoring program. The home visitor must obtain written consent from the parents for the child's participation in the program. It is important to explain, in nontechnical language, the purpose of the questionnaires and instructions for their completion.

It is also important for the parents to understand the role of the home visitor: to help parents complete the questionnaires, being as nondirective as possible, offering support, and helping to make the time enjoyable for the family. For optimal results, the home visitor should encourage maximum parental independence in completing the questionnaires, providing assistance when necessary, answering questions, and using the time for communication about the child's development.

Ideally, questionnaires should be mailed 1–2 weeks before the scheduled home visit to give parents the opportunity to observe their child's skills over time. Program staff should assemble needed ASQ materials for completion of questionnaires. A complete list of materials can be found in Appendix E. Upon completion and review of the questionnaire, the home visitor may choose to score the questionnaire with the parents, offering information and feedback or making appropriate referrals. The home visitor may offer activities that encourage positive parent–child interaction, while promoting optimal development. Intervention activities, contained in Appendix D, may be suggested during the home visit, or the Intervention Activities Sheets can be left with the parents for use until the next visit. The home visitor also may leave the current questionnaire and/or the subsequent questionnaire with the family so they can observe their child's development over the next 4–6 months.

As mentioned previously, the Information Summary Sheet, provided on the last page of each questionnaire, can be used on the home visit. This sheet allows the parents to score the questionnaire independently or with assistance from the home visitor. Scoring the questionnaire with the parents allows immediate feedback and follow-up, if necessary. The following list details the steps and decisions involved in implementing the ASQ system while on a home visit. In addition, a videotape, *The Ages & Stages Questionnaires on a Home Visit* (Farrell & Potter, 1995), is available.

1. Obtain consent from the parent(s) to participate in the monitoring program.
2. Telephone and schedule a home visit date and time. Photocopy the language-appropriate (English or Spanish) and age-appropriate questionnaires. Arrange for an interpreter if necessary.
3. Mail the age-appropriate questionnaire to the child's home 2 weeks before the visit. Use the questionnaire appropriate for the child's age. Questionnaires can be completed up to 1 month before and after the child's corresponding chronological age, creating a 2-month "window" for the use of each questionnaire. If the child's age falls outside of the 2-month "window" at the time of the home visit, give the parents the previous age interval questionnaire to complete. The next questionnaire interval can be left with the parents or mailed 1 or 2 weeks before the interval date.
4. Assemble appropriate toys and materials needed to complete the questionnaire. A complete list of materials can be found in Appendix E. Review each questionnaire carefully to know what toys and materials to bring.

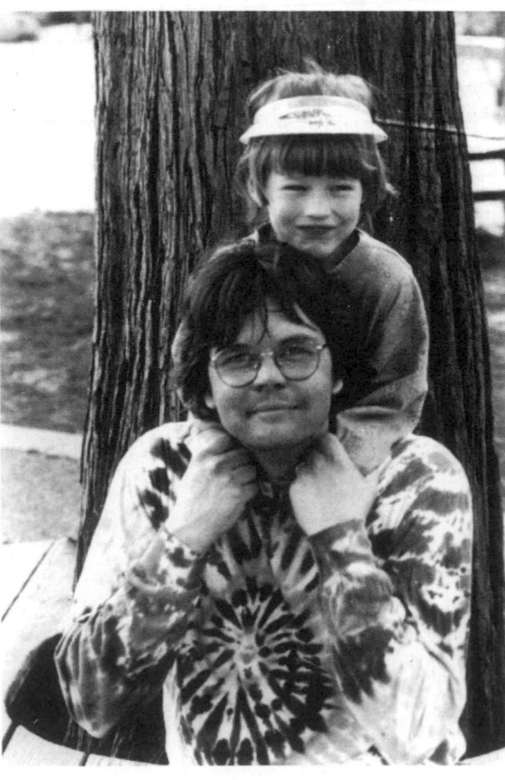

5. Determine whether the parents are capable of reading and comprehending the questionnaire.
   a. *For parents who are unable to read or are otherwise unable to complete the questionnaire* (e.g., as a result of mental illness, developmental disability, or a language difference):
      - The home visitor may read the items on the questionnaire.
      - The home visitor may demonstrate for parents how to elicit the behavior required for questionnaire items.
   b. *For parents who are able to read and comprehend the questionnaire:*
      - Parents can read and administer the questionnaire with the home visitor's assistance.
      - The home visitor may demonstrate how to elicit the behaviors required for questionnaire completion.

6. To describe the questionnaire, the home visitor can give the following information:
   a. Description of the ASQ system as a tool parents can use to check their child's development
   b. Clarification of the home visitor's role (i.e., to read and demonstrate how to elicit desired behavior)
   c. Ideas for involving family members, including siblings, in the elicitation of behaviors described on the questionnaires
7. Begin the questionnaire by completing the second page (i.e., demographic information).
   a. In response to "Who is completing this questionnaire?" the home visitor's name should be entered if he or she is doing so.
8. Explain the scoring system.
   a. *Yes* indicates the child is performing the behavior.
   b. *Sometimes* indicates the child is just beginning to perform the behavior (i.e., it is an emerging skill).
   c. *Not yet* indicates the child is not yet performing the behavior.
9. Introduce each area of development on the questionnaire.
   a. *Communication* items focus on language skills—both what the child understands and what he or she can say.
   b. *Gross motor* items focus on large muscle movement and coordination.
   c. *Fine motor* items focus on small muscle movement and coordination.
   d. *Problem solving* items focus on the child's play with toys.
   e. *Personal-social* items focus on the child's interactions with toys and other children.
10. Administer the questionnaire.
    a. If necessary, read each item.
    b. Paraphrase items as needed for parents who seem to need clarification.
    c. When appropriate, rephrase questions in terms of the family's values or cultural orientation.
    d. Comment on the child's accomplishments whenever possible. Praise the child directly. Highlight the parents' strengths and reinforce positive parent–child interactions.
    e. Adapt materials used for questionnaire items to the family's culture and values (e.g., some cultures do not use mirrors).
    f. For items the parents cannot answer with certainty, have them try to elicit the behaviors while the home visitor is present.
    g. If the child is uncooperative and the parents are unsure whether the child can perform a behavior, the home visitor can call parents in 1–2 weeks, thereby giving the parents more time to try the item(s).
11. Complete the Overall section, paying close attention to the parents' concerns.
    a. Offer suggestions and resources when appropriate.
    b. Encourage dialogue about the child's development and parenting issues.
12. Score the questionnaire.
    a. The home visitor can do the scoring or show the parents how to do the scoring.
    b. Compare the child's area scores with the cutoff scores indicated on the Information Summary Sheet.

13. Discuss the results with the parents.
    a. Explain the area scores.
    b. Using the bar graph on the Information Summary Sheet, show the parents where the child's scores fall in relation to the cutoff scores.
    c. Encourage dialogue with the parents about the child's development.
    d. Discuss referral options if necessary.
14. Offer intervention activity suggestions (see Appendix D) appropriate to the child's current and upcoming questionnaire age interval.
    a. Describe some of the activities with the parents.
    b. Encourage the parents to place the activities in an accessible place (e.g., on refrigerator door).
15. If appropriate, leave the next *Ages & Stages Questionnaire* for the parent to monitor the child's growth and development during the next 2–6 months.
16. Make arrangements for follow-up, referral, or the next home visit.

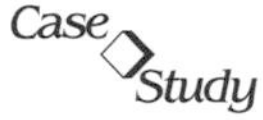

At least half of the families participating in Steps-Ahead have a home visitor help them complete the *Ages & Stages Questionnaires.* Although there is a diverse mix of parents who are assisted by home visitors, the most typical parent is single and unemployed. For most, transportation is difficult, and the parents appreciate the occasional company of another adult. Lonni and her baby, Amanda, were enrolled in Steps-Ahead 2 years ago when Amanda was born prematurely. Lonni was 16 years old at the time. She qualified for other programs that assisted her in finding housing and parenting support groups. Lonni and her social worker from Steps-Ahead have participated in several team meetings with other agencies to develop comprehensive goals and objectives for the family. When Lonni first began to complete the *Ages & Stages Questionnaires* with the social worker, she was skeptical and gave pat answers to many of the items. With time, the social worker was able to reassure Lonni and help build the confidence she needed to accurately observe and complete items on the questionnaires.

Procedures Involving Primary Health Care Providers For optimal results in a physician's or primary health care provider's office, it is suggested that the questionnaires be mailed to the parents' home at the designated age intervals (with the corrected age used when applicable). Parents can then complete the ASQ at home, trying each item with the child as necessary, and return the completed questionnaires to the provider's office or a central location. As an alternative, primary health care providers may mail a questionnaire 1–2 weeks before the child reaches the interval date (e.g., 8 or 12 months), and parents can bring the completed questionnaire to the office when the child is brought in for an appointment.

For parents who do not return the questionnaires and for parents with no permanent address, the questionnaires may be completed in the waiting room of a health care provider; a professional or other staff member may assist the parents as necessary. The ASQ materials list in Appendix E can be used to assemble needed toys and supplies for completion of the questionnaires. (As indicated previously, the *Ages & Stages Questionnaires* also can be completed by interview over the telephone or in person.)

Completing the ASQ in the waiting room is the least effective alternative for several reasons. First, objects (e.g., blocks, pencil and paper, a mirror) must be available so that parents can try the questionnaire items with their children. Second, parents may not have the time or attention necessary to complete the questionnaires in an office or clinic environment; similarly, the child may be uncooperative in the clinic environment. Third, it may be impossible to schedule an appointment to coincide with the questionnaire age intervals. Although questionnaires can be completed when the child is as much as 1 month older or younger than the age indicated on the questionnaire, it is sometimes difficult to arrange to see the parents during this "window" (see the discussion on Screening Children on Dates Between Questionnaire Age Intervals in the next section); failure to administer the questionnaire during the "window" can affect validity (see Appendix F).

Even with the availability of the optional questionnaires (i.e., 6, 10, 14, 18, 22, 27, 33, 42, 54 months), some children will have appointments that fall between designated age intervals. In these cases, it is suggested that the previous, or "younger," questionnaire be completed first. If the child does well with the items on this questionnaire, then the next ASQ age interval may be completed. If a child's performance falls below the cutoff point in any area, a duplicate questionnaire can be mailed or taken home to be completed at the next appropriate age interval. In situations like this, clinical judgment may be needed to evaluate the child's performance.

Case Study

Several pediatricians serve on the board of directors for the Steps-Ahead program. In particular, Dr. Bram found the *Ages & Stages Questionnaires* useful as a screening tool for his patients. Initially, he decided to try the questionnaires with a small number of patients, with the goal of adopting the ASQ system as his main developmental screening tool. Dr. Bram randomly selected 50 families with children between the ages of 1 month and 24 months. He sent a letter that described the ASQ system and the purpose of completing the questionnaires and that requested parents' permission to send them. Dr. Bram's office staff mailed the appropriate questionnaires using the mail-out procedures on pages 53–56. When parents brought their children to his office for well-child checkups, Dr. Bram reviewed the results of the questionnaires with the parents and answered questions as needed.

As part of his analysis of the ASQ system, Dr. Bram computed return rates and percentage of children needing referral; he also determined how parents felt about completing the questionnaires. His return rate averaged 80%, and the percentage of children needing referral (based on scores in one or more areas of development below the cutoff point) was 12%. Parents' responses during the well-child checkups indicated they felt the questionnaires were informative and easy to complete. Dr. Bram also felt the questionnaires gave parents a springboard from which they could ask questions about their child's development. After 1 year, Dr. Bram gave all the parents who brought their children to his practice the option of completing questionnaires prior to well-child visits.

Screening Children on Dates Between Questionnaire Age Intervals As discussed previously, because each questionnaire is valid for 1 month before and after the indicated age, there is a 2-month "window" for use. For example, a 12 month questionnaire can be used for children between 11 and 13 months of age. If a child's age falls outside of the 2-month "window," it may be useful to have the parents complete two questionnaires.

If, for instance, an infant is 44 months old, the parents may be asked to complete both the 42 and 48 month questionnaires. If the child successfully completes all of the items on the 42 month questionnaire, the 48 month questionnaire should be given. However, if the infant is unable to demonstrate most of the activities listed on the 42 month questionnaire, it is likely this child should be referred for further evaluation. When using questionnaires outside the "window," a professional with expertise in child development should exercise his or her judgment in the evaluation of the child's performance. The professional should bear in mind that the items in each developmental area are arranged in developmental order.

The more advanced, or "older," questionnaires also can be given to the parents to complete when the child reaches the next questionnaire age interval. Still another option is to telephone the parents on the second interval date (e.g., 48 months for the child discussed in the previous paragraph) to see if the child can successfully perform most of the items on the questionnaire.

Case Study

Steps-Ahead occasionally uses the *Ages & Stages Questionnaires* for children whose age falls outside the 2-month "window" for a specific questionnaire. This usually happens when the staff screen a child about whom they are concerned but do not anticipate seeing again (see the discussion of One-Time Screening Procedures on pp. 56–57).

Emily came to the attention of the Steps-Ahead staff when her mother, Ann, began to attend a drug treatment program. Emily was 39 months old and remained with Ann while Ann was in the residential treatment program. The staff at the treatment facility contacted Steps-Ahead with concerns about Emily's development. Because Ann's treatment was ending soon, the social worker at Steps-Ahead made a visit to the treatment facility and assisted Ann in completing the 36 and 42 month questionnaires. The social worker scored both questionnaires. Emily seemed to be developing typically according to her scores on the 36 month ASQ and was able to do a few items from each area on the 42 month ASQ. Ann had some concerns about Emily's language skills: Emily's communication scores were low but not below the cutoff point on the 36 month questionnaire. Following a discussion of options with Ann, the Steps-Ahead social worker decided that referral to a speech-language pathologist was in order. Ann signed a release of information form and was given a referral to have Emily's speech and language evaluated. The social worker gave the 36 and 42 month questionnaires back to Ann along with a copy of the Intervention Activities Sheet for 36- to 48-month-olds (see Appendix D). The social worker modeled games and activities related to the communication area.

Cultural and Language Adaptations The items on the *Ages & Stages Questionnaires* have been carefully selected, and, when possible, materials needed to complete the questionnaires are suggested. Although most parents will find the questionnaires easy to understand and use in the home environment, there may be situations in which the items are not appropriate for a given family, culture, or geographic area. For example, on the 8 month questionnaire, parents are asked whether their child pats a mirror. In some cultures, opportunities for mirror play are not provided. In these instances, the item may be omitted. (Directions for scoring questionnaires with missing responses are given on pp. 76–77.)

Sometimes families may not have access to certain materials and/or may not be familiar with certain objects or toys needed to complete items. In most of these situations, alternative materials may be substituted. However, it is important to examine the intent of the item to ensure that the adapted materials will adequately assess the skill under scrutiny. For example, in Hawaii, home visitors found that children rarely used zippered coats or jackets, making items requiring these materials difficult to observe. In order to assess these items, home visitors provided a large purse with a zipper that could be substituted for the zippered coat. If substitutions cannot be made, it is recommended that the item be omitted and the questionnaire scored using the directions provided for missing responses on pages 76–77.

Determining when to make cultural adaptations may be difficult. As mentioned previously, there are times when items will have to be omitted because they are not culturally appropriate. Before the questionnaires are given to some families, it may be best to consult someone from the specific culture who has experience working with children and families; this is especially relevant when a translator is needed.

Another option when materials and equipment are not available is to encourage parents to look for objects outside the home. Many parks, child care centers, and schoolyards may have the needed objects. For example, in the southwestern United States, many homes are built without stairs. To complete gross motor items involving stairs, parents may be directed to playground equipment in a local park or building.

When a child's native language is not English, it is recommended that questionnaires be administered in the primary language spoken in the home. Spanish, French, and Korean translations of the questionnaires are available. If the primary language spoken in the home is not English or one of these other languages, a translator may be required. When a translator is needed to complete the questionnaires with the family, he or she must be adequately trained in child development. The translator must have a thorough understanding of the intent of each item on the questionnaire. Translators should receive training on the use of the questionnaires, along with consistent directions for translating items. If more than one translator from a particular culture is working for the program, it is especially important that agreement about translation be established. It is also important that words that are requested on the questionnaires, such as "mama" or "dada," are translated appropriately.

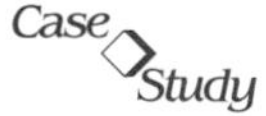

Several families who have recently immigrated to the United States have been referred to the Steps-Ahead program. For the most part, these families share common values concerning child development. However, for a few families, strong beliefs against putting children on the floor to play until a certain age preclude the completion of many of the gross motor items on the ASQ. The Steps-Ahead social worker asked these parents if they could try some of the items on a table or bed. This adaptation seemed to work. The values of the families were respected, and at the same time information about the child's developmental progress was obtained.

Score the Questionnaires

As described previously, each questionnaire contains 30 items that cover five developmental areas and an additional set of general questions about the child's overall health and development. Each developmental area contains six items; each area has an approximate developmental quotient range between 75 and 100. The rationale for selecting this restricted range is that children who are performing above 100 are probably developing without problems, while children scoring below 75 may have significant problems. Scoring procedures depend on whether all of the questionnaire items are answered or some are left unanswered; each procedure is described next. First, however, a general discussion of scoring the developmental sections and evaluating the Overall section is provided; the use of the cutoff bar graphs on the Information Summary Sheet is addressed as well. Scoring procedures are discussed further in the videotape *ASQ Scoring & Referral.*

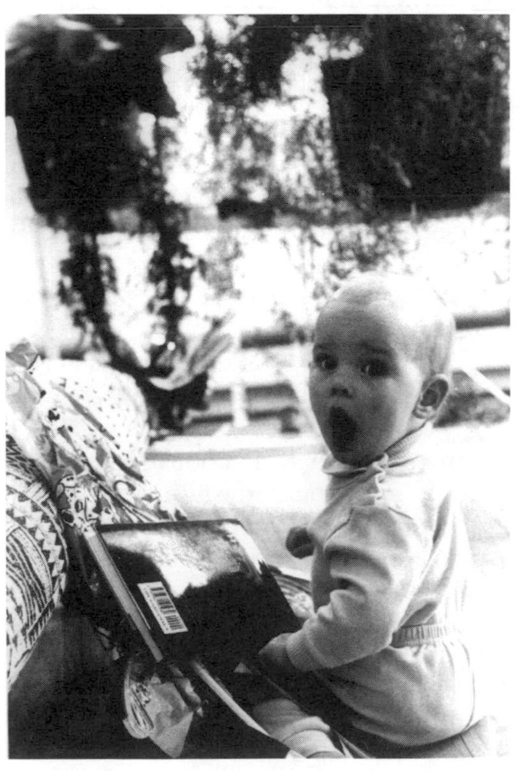

Developmental Area Items For each questionnaire item, a score line is provided to the right of the boxes. Parents check *yes, sometimes,* or *not yet* (see Figure 16). The scoring system allows 10 points for each *yes,* 5 points for each *sometimes,* and 0 points for each *not yet.* These scores may be recorded on the score lines. On a few of the questionnaires, there are items that ask about behaviors the child may have performed at one time but no longer does because he or she has acquired more advanced skills (e.g., crawling replaced by walking). On these questionnaires, parents are instructed to answer *yes* to items their child performed earlier but no longer does. If parents mistakenly answer *not yet* or *sometimes* to an easier item (e.g., pertaining to crawling) but *yes* to a more advanced item (e.g., pertaining to walking), the score for the earlier item should be changed to 10 (for a *yes* response) before computing the total area score. Items relating to more advanced behaviors that should be changed are indicated in the scoring instructions on each questionnaire.

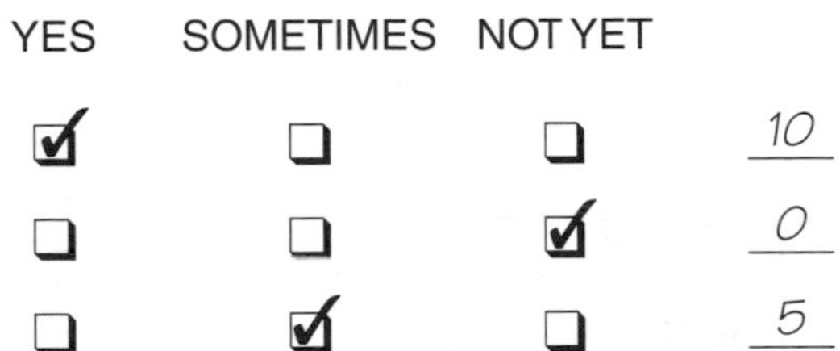

YES	SOMETIMES	NOT YET	
☑	☐	☐	10
☐	☐	☑	0
☐	☑	☐	5

Figure 16. A score line is provided for each questionnaire item. The person scoring the questionnaire should enter 10 for *yes* responses, 5 for *sometimes* responses, and 0 for *not yet* responses.

Total scores for each developmental area may be recorded on the line located below the last item in each area (see Figure 17). To score the developmental areas, first, all of the *yes* and *sometimes* responses can be added for each area. The scores can then be compared to the established cutoffs indicated on the Information Summary Sheet to determine whether the child's performance meets the criteria for referral. Children whose scores are above the cutoff points are not identified as needing further assessment or are considered to be developing typically. Children whose scores fall on or below the cutoff scores are "identified," or considered to be in need of follow-up and should be referred for further assessment.

Case Study

Sam Fuller was chronologically 5 months old when the 4 month ASQ was completed by his parents, Joyce and Bill Fuller. Because Sam was born 4 weeks prematurely, Steps-Ahead corrected his birthdate for prematurity. Joyce and Bill adopted Sam when he was 2 weeks old; Sam's birth mother had received no prenatal care during the pregnancy. Sam's birth weight was low for his gestational age, and he tested positive for drug exposure. He

YES	SOMETIMES	NOT YET	
☑	☐	☐	10
☑	☐	☐	10
☐	☑	☐	5
☑	☐	☐	10
☐	☐	☑	0
☐	☐	☑	0
		COMMUNICATION TOTAL	35

Figure 17. The child's scores for each item should be totaled by developmental area. Totals should be recorded on the indicated lines for easy translation to the bar graphs on the Information Summary Sheet.

was hospitalized for 2 weeks with newborn tremors, hypertonia, and respiratory distress. As shown in Figure 18, all of Sam's scores on the 4 month ASQ were low, with the gross motor total falling below the cutoff point. In the Overall section Joyce and Bill commented that Sam stands on his toes (rather than flat on his feet), doesn't sleep at night, and cries a lot. Given the low scores and the concerns noted by Sam's parents, the Steps-Ahead social worker is recommending further evaluation, with special attention to Sam's motor abilities.

Delia Conley was born 4 months ago to Janice Conley. There were no problems at birth, and Delia's birth weight and other medical characteristics were typical. Delia and her family qualified for participation in Steps-Ahead because Janice was 19 at the time of Delia's birth, and she had not completed high school. Janice also has another child, Jamie, who is 2 years old. Delia's scores on the ASQ (see Figure 19) are well above the cutoff points in all areas, and Janice did not list any concerns in the Overall section. Steps-Ahead will continue to monitor Delia's development, mailing the 8 month questionnaire in approximately 4 months.

For a child whose scores on a questionnaire fall just above the cutoff point in one or more areas, a follow-up contact with the parents is recommended. This follow-up contact consists of a telephone call or visit to talk about items not yet scored and discuss any parental concerns. This child may continue to be monitored using the *Ages & Stages Questionnaires* or may be referred for assessment, depending on the parents' concerns and information. If several areas of development receive scores that are low but not below the cutoff points, the child may need to be referred for assessment. In this case, it is important to contact parents to discuss the results and possible referral.

Regardless of a child's scores, when a parent records a concern in the Overall section of the questionnaire, program staff should respond. For example, a child may miss many of the expressive items in the communication area on the 16 month ASQ and still not receive scores that fall below the cutoff point. If, however, the parents have noted a concern in response to the question, "Do you think your child talks like other toddlers his [or her] age?" in the Overall section, the possibility of a referral for further assessment should be discussed with the parents.

Overall Section The Overall section, which contains questions such as "Do you think your child hears well?" and "Does anything about your child worry you?" is not scored but should serve as a general indicator of parental concerns. This section is important because parents may indicate a concern that is not addressed in the developmental areas of the questionnaire. Parents answer these questions by checking *yes* or *no,* and when appropriate explaining the response.

On the 4, 6, 8, 10, and 12 month questionnaires, the Overall section includes questions about whether the child uses both hands equally well and stands flat on surfaces most of the time. These questions are included as a means of detecting cerebral palsy. A *no* answer to either of these questions indicates that a follow-up telephone call or visit is necessary. In general, any concern about development noted by the parents in the Overall section should be discussed with parents, and a referral made if appropriate.

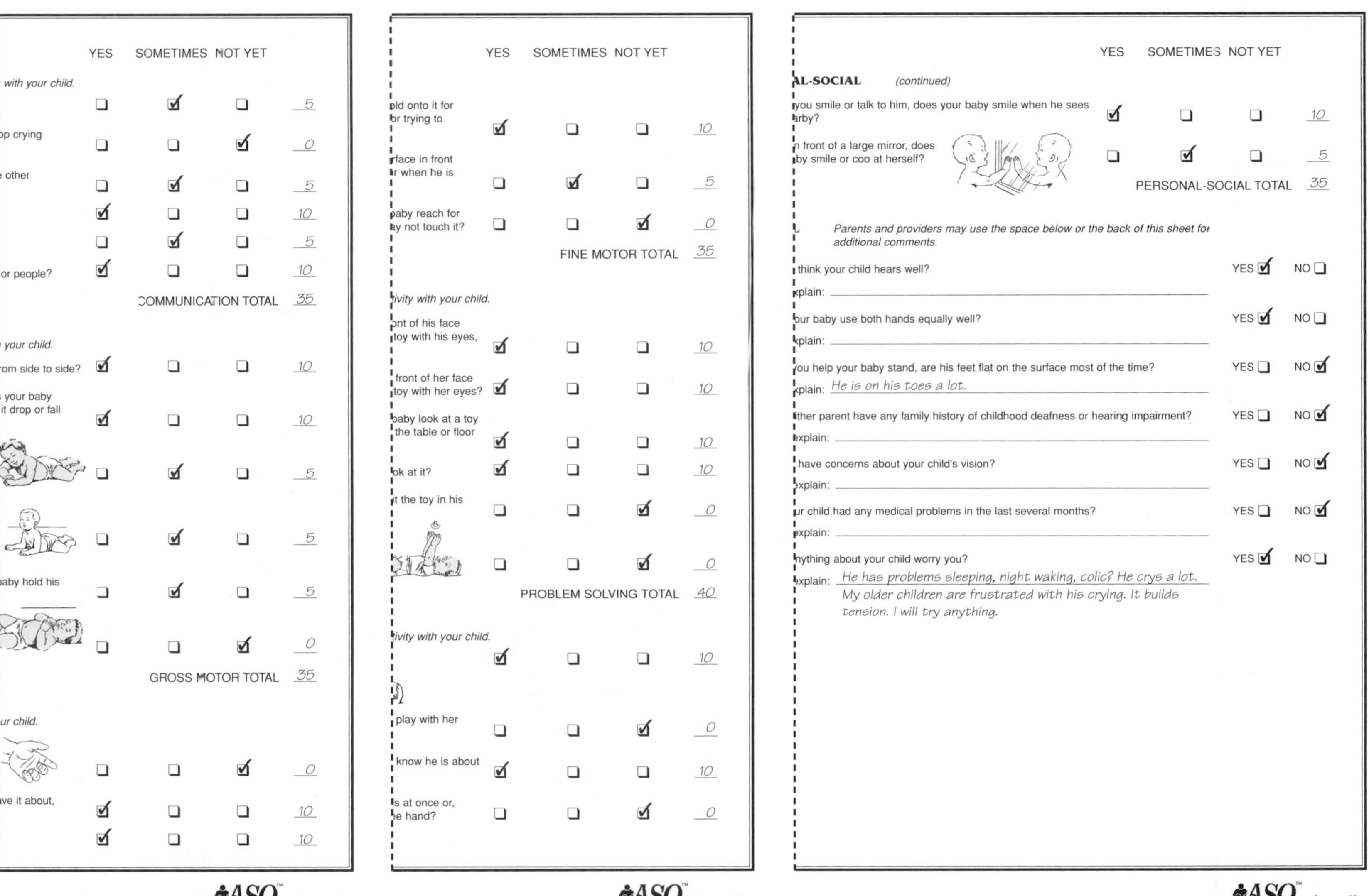

	YES	SOMETIMES	NOT YET	
with your child.				
	☐	☑	☐	5
op crying	☐	☐	☑	0
e other	☐	☑	☐	5
	☑	☐	☐	10
	☐	☑	☐	5
or people?	☑	☐	☐	10
		COMMUNICATION TOTAL		35
your child.				
rom side to side?	☑	☐	☐	10
your baby it drop or fall	☑	☐	☐	10
	☐	☑	☐	5
	☐	☑	☐	5
aby hold his	☐	☑	☐	5
	☐	☐	☑	0
		GROSS MOTOR TOTAL		35
ur child.				
	☐	☐	☑	0
ve it about,	☑	☐	☐	10
	☑	☐	☐	10

ASQ™ 4 months

	YES	SOMETIMES	NOT YET	
old onto it for or trying to	☑	☐	☐	10
face in front r when he is	☐	☑	☐	5
aby reach for y not touch it?	☐	☐	☑	0
		FINE MOTOR TOTAL		35
ivity with your child.				
ont of his face toy with his eyes,	☑	☐	☐	10
front of her face toy with her eyes?	☑	☐	☐	10
aby look at a toy the table or floor	☑	☐	☐	10
ok at it?	☑	☐	☐	10
t the toy in his	☐	☐	☑	0
	☐	☐	☑	0
		PROBLEM SOLVING TOTAL		40
ivity with your child.				
	☑	☐	☐	10
play with her	☐	☐	☑	0
know he is about	☑	☐	☐	10
s at once or, e hand?	☐	☐	☑	0

ASQ™ 4 months

AL-SOCIAL *(continued)*

	YES	SOMETIMES	NOT YET	
you smile or talk to him, does your baby smile when he sees arby?	☑	☐	☐	10
n front of a large mirror, does by smile or coo at herself?	☐	☑	☐	5
		PERSONAL-SOCIAL TOTAL		35

Parents and providers may use the space below or the back of this sheet for additional comments.

think your child hears well?	YES ☑	NO ☐
xplain:		
our baby use both hands equally well?	YES ☑	NO ☐
xplain:		
ou help your baby stand, are his feet flat on the surface most of the time?	YES ☐	NO ☑
xplain: *He is on his toes a lot.*		
ther parent have any family history of childhood deafness or hearing impairment?	YES ☐	NO ☑
xplain:		
have concerns about your child's vision?	YES ☐	NO ☑
xplain:		
ur child had any medical problems in the last several months?	YES ☐	NO ☑
xplain:		
nything about your child worry you?	YES ☑	NO ☐
xplain: *He has problems sleeping, night waking, colic? He crys a lot. My older children are frustrated with his crying. It builds tension. I will try anything.*		

ASQ™ 4 months

continued

Figure 18. The scoring sections of Sam Fuller's 4 month ASQ revealed low scores in each of the developmental areas, with gross motor falling below the cutoff point. His parents also indicated concerns in the Overall section. Based on these results, the social worker who scored the questionnaire is recommending further evaluation (see next page).

Figure 18. (continued)

4 Month ASQ Information Summary

Child's name: *Sam Fuller*

Person filling out the ASQ: *Joyce and Bill Fuller*

Mailing address: *2198 Cherry Lane*

Telephone:

Today's date: *September 20, 1998*

Date of birth: *April 24, 1998*

Corrected date of birth: *May 24, 1998*

Relationship to child: *Mom and Dad*

City: *Cottage Grove* State: *OR* ZIP: *97472*

Assisting in ASQ completion:

OVERALL: Please transfer the answers in the Overall section of the questionnaire by circling "yes" or "no" and reporting any comments.

1. Hears well? (YES) NO
   Comments:
2. Uses both hands equally well? (YES) NO
   Comments:
3. Baby's feet flat on the surface? YES (NO)
   Comments: *He is on his toes a lot.*
4. Family history of hearing impairment? YES (NO)
   Comments:
5. Vision concerns? YES (NO)
   Comments:
6. Recent medical problems? YES (NO)
   Comments:
7. Other concerns? (YES) NO
   Comments: *not sleeping and crying a lot*

SCORING THE QUESTIONNAIRE

1. Be sure each item has been answered. If an item cannot be answered, refer to the ratio scoring procedure in *The ASQ User's Guide.*
2. Score each item on the questionnaire by writing the appropriate number on the line by each item answer.
   YES = 10 SOMETIMES = 5 NOT YET = 0
3. Add up the item scores for each area and record these totals in the space provided for area totals.
4. Indicate the child's total score for each area by filling in the appropriate circle on the chart below. For example, if the total score for the Communication area was 50, fill in the circle below 50 in the first row.

Total	0	5	10	15	20	25	30	35	40	45	50	55	60
Communication	○	○	○	○	○	○	○	●	○	○	○	○	○
Gross motor	○	○	○	○	○	○	○	●	○	○	○	○	○
Fine motor	○	○	○	○	○	○	○	●	○	○	○	○	○
Problem solving	○	○	○	○	○	○	○	○	●	○	○	○	○
Personal-social	○	○	○	○	○	○	○	●	○	○	○	○	○
Total	0	5	10	15	20	25	30	35	40	45	50	55	60

Examine the blackened circles for each area in the chart above.

5. If the child's total score falls within the ▭ area, the child appears to be doing well in this area at this time.
6. If the child's total score falls within the ▬ area, talk with a professional. The child may need further evaluation.

OPTIONAL: The specific answers to each item on the questionnaire can be recorded below on the summary chart.

4 months	Score	Cutoff
Communication	*35*	33.3
Gross motor	*35*	40.1
Fine motor	*35*	27.5
Problem solving	*40*	35.0
Personal-social	*35*	33.0

Item	Communication Y	S	N	Gross motor Y	S	N	Fine motor Y	S	N	Problem solving Y	S	N	Personal-social Y	S	N
1	○	●	○	●	○	○	○	○	●	●	○	○	●	○	○
2	○	○	●	●	●	○	●	○	○	●	○	○	○	○	●
3	○	●	○	○	●	○	●	○	○	●	○	○	●	○	○
4	●	○	○	○	●	○	●	○	○	●	○	○	○	○	●
5	○	●	○	○	○	○	○	●	○	○	○	●	●	○	○
6	●	○	○	○	○	●	○	○	●	○	○	●	○	●	○

Administering program or provider: *STEPS-AHEAD*

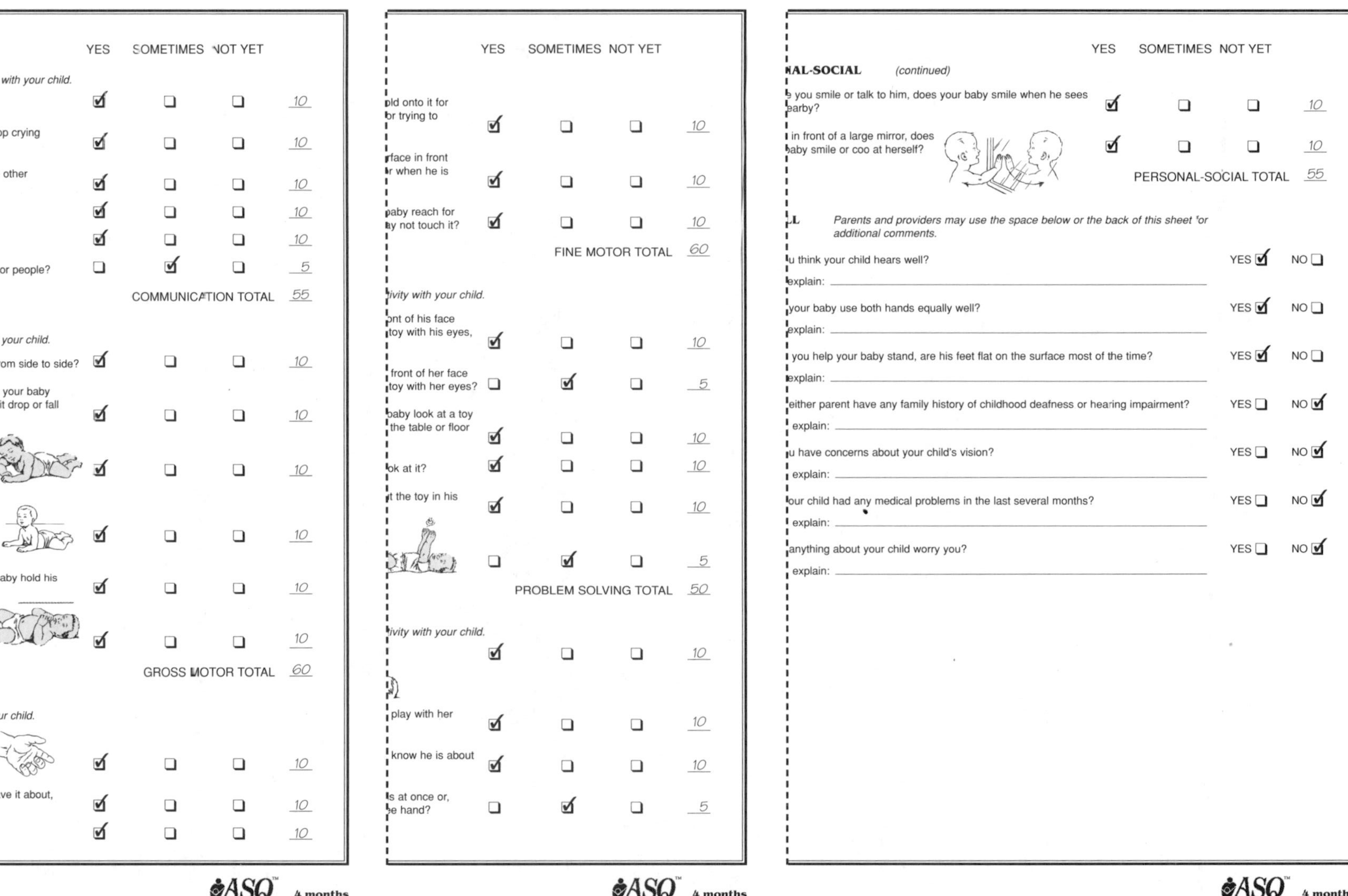

	YES	SOMETIMES	NOT YET	
...with your child.				
	✓			10
...op crying	✓			10
...e other	✓			10
	✓			10
	✓			10
...or people?		✓		5
COMMUNICATION TOTAL				55
...your child.				
...rom side to side?	✓			10
...s your baby ...it drop or fall	✓			10
	✓			10
	✓			10
...aby hold his	✓			10
	✓			10
GROSS MOTOR TOTAL				60
...ur child.				
	✓			10
...ave it about,	✓			10
	✓			10

ASQ™ 4 months

	YES	SOMETIMES	NOT YET	
...ld onto it for ...r trying to	✓			10
...face in front ...r when he is	✓			10
...aby reach for ...y not touch it?	✓			10
FINE MOTOR TOTAL				60
...ivity with your child.				
...nt of his face ...toy with his eyes,	✓			10
...front of her face ...toy with her eyes?		✓		5
...aby look at a toy ...the table or floor	✓			10
...k at it?	✓			10
...t the toy in his	✓			10
		✓		5
PROBLEM SOLVING TOTAL				50
...ivity with your child.				
	✓			10
...play with her	✓			10
...know he is about	✓			10
...s at once or, ...e hand?		✓		5

ASQ™ 4 months

...AL-SOCIAL *(continued)*

	YES	SOMETIMES	NOT YET	
...e you smile or talk to him, does your baby smile when he sees ...earby?	✓			10
...in front of a large mirror, does ...aby smile or coo at herself?	✓			10
PERSONAL-SOCIAL TOTAL				55

...L *Parents and providers may use the space below or the back of this sheet for additional comments.*

	YES	NO
...u think your child hears well?	✓	
...your baby use both hands equally well?	✓	
...you help your baby stand, are his feet flat on the surface most of the time?	✓	
...either parent have any family history of childhood deafness or hearing impairment?		✓
...u have concerns about your child's vision?		✓
...our child had any medical problems in the last several months?		✓
...anything about your child worry you?		✓

explain: (blank after each question)

ASQ™ 4 months

continued

Figure 19. Delia Conley's scores on the 4 month ASQ indicated typical development, and her mother had not listed any concerns in the Overall section. Steps-Ahead will continue to monitor Delia's developmental progress.

Figure 19. (continued)

4 Month ASQ Information Summary

Child's name: Delia Conley
Person filling out the ASQ: Janice Conley
Mailing address: 39078 Lana Ave.
Telephone:
Today's date: November 4, 1998

Date of birth: July 4, 1998
Corrected date of birth:
Relationship to child: Mother
City: Eugene State: OR ZIP: 97402
Assisting in ASQ completion:

OVERALL: Please transfer the answers in the Overall section of the questionnaire by circling "yes" or "no" and reporting any comments.

1. Hears well? (YES) NO
   Comments:
2. Uses both hands equally well? (YES) NO
   Comments:
3. Baby's feet flat on the surface? (YES) NO
   Comments:
4. Family history of hearing impairment? YES (NO)
   Comments:
5. Vision concerns? YES (NO)
   Comments:
6. Recent medical problems? YES (NO)
   Comments:
7. Other concerns? YES (NO)
   Comments:

SCORING THE QUESTIONNAIRE

1. Be sure each item has been answered. If an item cannot be answered, refer to the ratio scoring procedure in *The ASQ User's Guide.*
2. Score each item on the questionnaire by writing the appropriate number on the line by each item answer.
   YES = 10 SOMETIMES = 5 NOT YET = 0
3. Add up the item scores for each area and record these totals in the space provided for area totals.
4. Indicate the child's total score for each area by filling in the appropriate circle on the chart below. For example, if the total score for the Communication area was 50, fill in the circle below 50 in the first row.

Total	0	5	10	15	20	25	30	35	40	45	50	55	60
Communication	○	○	○	○	○	○	○	○	○	○	○	●	○
Gross motor	○	○	○	○	○	○	○	○	○	○	○	○	●
Fine motor	○	○	○	○	○	○	○	○	○	○	○	○	●
Problem solving	○	○	○	○	○	○	○	○	○	○	●	○	○
Personal-social	○	○	○	○	○	○	○	○	○	○	○	●	○
Total	0	5	10	15	20	25	30	35	40	45	50	55	60

Examine the blackened circles for each area in the chart above.

5. If the child's total score falls within the ▭ area, the child appears to be doing well in this area at this time.
6. If the child's total score falls within the ▬ area, talk with a professional. The child may need further evaluation.

OPTIONAL: The specific answers to each item on the questionnaire can be recorded below on the summary chart.

4 months	Score	Cutoff
Communication	55	33.3
Gross motor	60	40.1
Fine motor	60	27.5
Problem solving	50	35.0
Personal-social	55	33.0

Item	Communication (Y S N)	Gross motor (Y S N)	Fine motor (Y S N)	Problem solving (Y S N)	Personal-social (Y S N)
1	● ○ ○	● ○ ○	● ○ ○	● ○ ○	● ○ ○
2	● ○ ○	● ○ ○	● ○ ○	○ ● ○	● ○ ○
3	● ○ ○	● ○ ○	● ○ ○	● ○ ○	● ○ ○
4	● ○ ○	● ○ ○	● ○ ○	● ○ ○	○ ● ○
5	● ○ ○	● ○ ○	● ○ ○	● ○ ○	● ○ ○
6	○ ● ○	● ○ ○	● ○ ○	○ ● ○	● ○ ○

Administering program or provider: STEPS-AHEAD

6

ASQ™ 4 months

Cutoff Points As mentioned above, the ASQ system uses cutoff points to determine whether a child's score on a questionnaire indicates that the child should be referred for an in-depth evaluation. The cutoff points have been generated for each area of development on each questionnaire based on more than 7,900 completed questionnaires. The cutoff points were derived by subtracting 2 standard deviations from the mean for each area of development (e.g., fine motor). (The communication areas on the 14, 16, 18, 20, 22, 24, 27, 30, and 33 month questionnaires were initially excepted from this guideline. For these cutoff scores, one item [10 points] was added.) Therefore, the mean for each area represents the average performance of a large number of children. The standard deviation represents the amount of variance for each mean score, or how much scores are likely to vary in a particular area. The cutoff points listed in Table 4 were generated to minimize the percentage of children overreferred and underreferred.[2] The cutoff points vary by area of development and by questionnaire interval. Appendix F at the end of this volume provides a more thorough discussion of the analyses used to balance the percentage of overreferral and underreferral based on the cutoff points.

It is possible for programs using the ASQ system to adjust the cutoff points they use, although this adjustment should be made thoughtfully. Chapter 4 provides a discussion of the basis on which programs may choose to adjust cutoff points. To adjust a cutoff point, the standard deviation is subtracted from the mean for each developmental area using the means and standard deviations provided in Table 3 on page 41. This number is then multiplied by 10 (to eliminate calculations using decimal points). For example, a program may choose to adopt a cutoff point that represents 1 standard deviation from the mean. One standard deviation would then be subtracted from the mean area scores.

Mean area score – standard deviation x 10 = cutoff score

For the communication area on the 8 month ASQ, the standard deviation of .86 would be subtracted from the area mean, 5.35, and multiplied by 10, resulting in a new cutoff point of 44.9.

$$5.35 - .86 = 4.49 \times 10 = 44.9$$

Programs that use this strategy should be aware that by changing the cutoff points, one also changes the sensitivity, specificity, overreferral and underreferral rates, and other related variables. Table 20 in Appendix F at the end of this guide provides the sensitivity, specificity, true positive, false positive, and overreferral and underreferral rates when the cutoff points are adjusted.

Scoring Complete Questionnaires When parents have answered the items on a questionnaire, the following scoring steps should be used:

1. Review the questionnaire for unanswered items. If all items are answered, proceed to Step 2. If any questions were left unanswered, try to contact the parents to score unanswered questions. If this is not possible, see the procedures outlined in the next section for Scoring Questionnaires with Unanswered Items.
2. Correct items marked *not yet* or *sometimes* if more advanced items are scored *yes*. (There are reminders on the questionnaires to do this where necessary.)

[2]In 2004, the cutoff scores for nine intervals were updated. These cutoff scores are shown in Table 4, appear in the fifth and later printings of the English and Spanish ASQ, and also apply to the French ASQ. The revised cutoff scores are also posted at http://www.brookespublishing.com/asqupdate. When the cutoff scores were updated, the 27 and 33 month communication area cutoffs were calculated by subtracting 2 standard deviations from the mean.

Table 4. Cutoff points by questionnaire interval and area of development

Questionnaire interval	Area of development	Cutoff point
4	Communication	33.3
	Gross motor	40.1
	Fine motor	27.5
	Problem solving	35.0
	Personal-social	33.0
6[a]	Communication	29.0
	Gross motor	19.5
	Fine motor	27.5
	Problem solving	37.0
	Personal-social	27.5
8	Communication	36.7
	Gross motor	24.3
	Fine motor	36.8
	Problem solving	32.3
	Personal-social	30.5
10[a]	Communication	25.0
	Gross motor	17.5
	Fine motor	39.0
	Problem solving	30.5
	Personal-social	30.0
12	Communication	15.8
	Gross motor	18.0
	Fine motor	28.4
	Problem solving	25.2
	Personal-social	20.1
14[a]	Communication	31.0[b]
	Gross motor	24.0
	Fine motor	25.0
	Problem solving	28.5
	Personal-social	22.5
16	Communication	34.5[b]
	Gross motor	32.3
	Fine motor	30.6
	Problem solving	26.9
	Personal-social	26.7
18[a]	Communication	23.0[b]
	Gross motor	41.5
	Fine motor	39.5
	Problem solving	33.0
	Personal-social	37.0
20	Communication	36.3[b]
	Gross motor	36.2
	Fine motor	39.8
	Problem solving	29.9
	Personal-social	35.2

(continued)

[a]In 2004, cutoff scores for these nine intervals were revised. The revised cutoff scores appear in this table and in the fifth and subsequent printings of the English and Spanish ASQ questionnaires and also apply to the French ASQ. The revised cutoff scores are also posted on-line at http://www.brookespublishing.com/asqupdates/

[b]Ten points (one item) have been added to these cutoffs in order to ensure that a child can successfully do at least one expressive item in the communication area.

[c]These cutoff points were adjusted using a statistical technique (receiver operating characteristic or ROC) to ensure best fit in terms of sensitivity and specificity.

Table 4. *(continued)*

Questionnaire interval	Area of development	Cutoff point
22	Communication	35.0[b]
	Gross motor	40.0
	Fine motor	36.5
	Problem solving	36.5
	Personal-social	39.5
24	Communication	36.5[b]
	Gross motor	36.0
	Fine motor	36.4
	Problem solving	32.9
	Personal-social	35.6
27[a]	Communication	33.5[b]
	Gross motor	35.0
	Fine motor	26.0
	Problem solving	37.0
	Personal-social	33.0
30	Communication	38.8
	Gross motor	30.6
	Fine motor	25.2
	Problem solving	28.9
	Personal-social	36.9
33[a]	Communication	35.0[b]
	Gross motor	41.5
	Fine motor	29.0
	Problem solving	36.5
	Personal-social	36.0
36	Communication	38.7
	Gross motor	35.7
	Fine motor	30.7
	Problem solving	38.6
	Personal-social	38.7
42[a]	Communication	38.0[b]
	Gross motor	45.0
	Fine motor	40.0
	Problem solving	39.0
	Personal-social	42.5
48	Communication	39.1
	Gross motor	32.9
	Fine motor	30.0[c]
	Problem solving	35.0[c]
	Personal-social	23.4
54[a]	Communication	50.0[b]
	Gross motor	42.5
	Fine motor	26.5
	Problem solving	33.0
	Personal-social	36.5
60	Communication	31.7
	Gross motor	32.7
	Fine motor	30.5
	Problem solving	30.1
	Personal-social	39.5

3. Score each item on the questionnaire using the following values:
   - *Yes* = 10 points
   - *Sometimes* = 5 points
   - *Not yet* = 0 points
4. Total the points in each area.
5. Plot the area totals on the bar graph provided on the Information Summary Sheet.
6. Note any area score(s) falling in the shaded portion of the bar graph. The child may require further assessment in these areas.
7. Read the responses in the Overall section carefully. Contact the parents for clarification if the answers suggest potential problems. Transfer the *yes* and *no* responses, along with comments when they are relevant, to the top portion of the Information Summary Sheet.

Scoring Questionnaires with Unanswered Items Occasionally, a parent does not provide answers to all of the items on a questionnaire. If this occurs, attempts should be made to contact the parent as soon as possible to obtain response(s) to missing item(s). If the missing responses are provided, the scorer should follow the steps outlined in the previous section. Please note that a category cannot be accurately scored when more than 2 items are left unanswered.

Sometimes parents omit an item because they are unsure of how to respond or because they have a concern about the child's performance of the behavior. For these reasons, it is important to attempt to reach parents when items are left unanswered. If contacting the parent is not possible, a ratio score for the area(s) affected can be computed. Ratio scores are computed because they do not penalize the child for unanswered items. A ratio score is computed by dividing the area's total points by the number of items answered in that area.

Area total ÷ number of items answered = ratio score

This formula will yield a number between 0 and 10. The ratio score is then added to the area total score, resulting in the final area score, which will be compared to the cutoff points on the Information Summary Sheet.

Ratio score + previous total = final area score

For example, on a 4 month questionnaire, a parent answered five of the six items in the gross motor area: three items were answered *yes* (30 points accumulated), one item was answered *sometimes* (5 points), and one item was answered *not yet* (0 points). The child's total gross motor score is 35, which is then divided by 5 (the number of items answered in the area), yielding a ratio score of 7.

$$35 \div 5 = 7$$

The ratio score of 7 is added to the previous total of 35, for a final gross motor score of 42.

$$7 + 35 = 42$$

The 4 month Information Summary Sheet bar graph indicates a gross motor cutoff of 40.1, suggesting that the child is developing typically in the gross motor area.

If two items are not completed in an area, the same formula for computing ratio scores is used, except that the ratio score is doubled before being added to the total score. For example, on the 16 month questionnaire, a parent answered four of the six items in the problem solving area: two items were answered *yes* (20 points accumulated), one item was answered *sometimes* (5 points), and one item was answered *not yet* (0 points). The child's total problem solving score is 25, which is then divided by 4, yielding a ratio score of 6.25.

$$25 \div 4 = 6.25$$

The ratio score of 6.25 is then doubled and added to the previous total of 25, for a final problem solving score of 37.50.

$$12.50 + 25 = 37.50$$

The 16 month Information Summary Sheet bar graph indicates a problem solving cutoff of 26.9, suggesting that the child is developing typically in the problem solving area.

If more than two items are omitted in any area, that area should not be scored. Parents should be contacted to discuss the omissions and to obtain answers for the items.

The following is a list of steps for scoring questionnaires with unanswered items:

1. If possible, contact the parents to complete unanswered questions. If this is not possible, proceed to Step 2. If the items are scored, follow the instructions for Scoring Complete Questionnaires on pages 73–76.
2. Follow the procedures described on pages 66–68 for the developmental areas the parents have completed in full.
3. For the remaining incompletely answered developmental areas, calculate ratio scores.
   - Score the answered items (10, 5, or 0), and total these scores.
   - Divide the area score by the number of answered items.
4. If one item has been omitted, add the ratio score to the previous area total score to obtain the final area score. If two items have been omitted in one area, double the ratio score before adding it to the previous area total score.
5. Plot the developmental area totals, including the ratio-based final area score(s), on the bar graph provided on the Information Summary Sheet.
6. Note any developmental area score(s) falling in the shaded portion of the bar graph. The child may require further assessment in these areas.
7. Read the responses in the Overall section carefully. Contact the parents for clarification if the answers suggest potential problems. Transfer the *yes* and *no* responses, along with comments when they are relevant, to the top portion of the Information Summary Sheet.

Recording Individual Item Responses The grid at the bottom of the Information Summary Sheet provides space to record responses to individual questionnaire items, as well as area total scores. If program staff wish to return the questionnaires to parents, the Information Summary Sheet provides a one-page summary of all questionnaire information, including individual questionnaire item responses. This information may be valuable at a later time if staff must determine whether a child needs a more in-depth developmental evaluation. In addition, programs with the resources to mechanically scan questionnaire data may use the grids as computer-ready forms.

Determine Follow-Up

For Children Whose Scores Indicate Typical Development Most scored questionnaires will indicate that the child is developing without problems; that is, the child's totals in the developmental areas are above the cutoff points indicated on the Information Summary Sheet bar graph. For these children, a letter can be sent to parents explaining that their child appears to be developing without problems and also indicating when the next questionnaire will need to be completed. Figure 20 is a sample feedback letter to parents of children whose scores indicate they are developing without problems. A Spanish translation of this letter is provided in Appendix C.

For Children Whose Scores Indicate a Need for Further Assessment For children whose scores on a questionnaire meet the referral criteria defined during the planning stage of the ASQ process (see Chapter 4), some action should be taken. Available options include the following:

- *Refer* a child whose score in one or more developmental areas is below the established cutoff point (i.e., 2 standard deviations below the mean) for that questionnaire interval.
- *Follow up* with a child whose score in a particular area is close to the cutoff point.
- *Follow up* with a child whose scores are above the cutoff points for each area but whose parent has indicated a concern in the Overall section of the questionnaire.

All of the above criteria could suggest that a child be referred for diagnostic testing. However, the only time that referral is always indicated is when a child's questionnaire score falls below the cutoff point in any area. To help keep track of scores on the questionnaires, a Summary of Questionnaire Results Sheet is provided in Figure 21. This form provides an easy way to look at a child's borderline or below-cutoff scores across questionnaire age inter-

Dear [fill in parents' or guardians' names]:

Thank you for completing the *Ages & Stages Questionnaire* for your child. Your responses on the questionnaire show that your child's development appears to be progressing well.

Another questionnaire will be mailed to you in [fill in number here] months. Please remember again the importance of completing all items and of mailing the questionnaire back as soon as possible. Feel free to call if you have any questions. Thank you for your interest in our program.

Sincerely,

[fill in staff member's name]
[fill in program name]

Figure 20. A sample feedback letter to parents or guardians whose children's questionnaire scores indicate typical development. A Spanish translation of this letter is contained in Appendix C.

Summary of Questionnaire Results Sheet

Child's name ______________________ ID# __________ Date of birth __________

Purpose: The purpose of this form is to permit the consolidation of information from individual ASQs so children's performances can be monitored over time.

Directions: Transfer item responses *(yes, sometimes, not yet)* from the questionnaire to the circles located in each rectangular box that correspond with each area. Parent concerns or other comments can be recorded in the Comments section.

Date completed __________

4 months	Score	Cutoff
Communication		33.3
Gross motor		40.1
Fine motor		27.5
Problem solving		35.0
Personal-social		33.0

	Communication			Gross motor			Fine motor			Problem solving			Personal-social		
	Y	S	N	Y	S	N	Y	S	N	Y	S	N	Y	S	N
1	○	○	○	○	○	○	○	○	○	○	○	○	○	○	○
2	○	○	○	○	○	○	○	○	○	○	○	○	○	○	○
3	○	○	○	○	○	○	○	○	○	○	○	○	○	○	○
4	○	○	○	○	○	○	○	○	○	○	○	○	○	○	○
5	○	○	○	○	○	○	○	○	○	○	○	○	○	○	○
6	○	○	○	○	○	○	○	○	○	○	○	○	○	○	○

Comments:

Date completed __________

6 months	Score	Cutoff
Communication		29.0
Gross motor		19.5
Fine motor		27.5
Problem solving		37.0
Personal-social		27.5

	Communication			Gross motor			Fine motor			Problem solving			Personal-social		
	Y	S	N	Y	S	N	Y	S	N	Y	S	N	Y	S	N
1	○	○	○	○	○	○	○	○	○	○	○	○	○	○	○
2	○	○	○	○	○	○	○	○	○	○	○	○	○	○	○
3	○	○	○	○	○	○	○	○	○	○	○	○	○	○	○
4	○	○	○	○	○	○	○	○	○	○	○	○	○	○	○
5	○	○	○	○	○	○	○	○	○	○	○	○	○	○	○
6	○	○	○	○	○	○	○	○	○	○	○	○	○	○	○

Comments:

Date completed __________

8 months	Score	Cutoff
Communication		36.7
Gross motor		24.3
Fine motor		36.8
Problem solving		32.3
Personal-social		30.5

	Communication			Gross motor			Fine motor			Problem solving			Personal-social		
	Y	S	N	Y	S	N	Y	S	N	Y	S	N	Y	S	N
1	○	○	○	○	○	○	○	○	○	○	○	○	○	○	○
2	○	○	○	○	○	○	○	○	○	○	○	○	○	○	○
3	○	○	○	○	○	○	○	○	○	○	○	○	○	○	○
4	○	○	○	○	○	○	○	○	○	○	○	○	○	○	○
5	○	○	○	○	○	○	○	○	○	○	○	○	○	○	○
6	○	○	○	○	○	○	○	○	○	○	○	○	○	○	○

Comments:

(continued)

Figure 21. The Summary of Questionnaire Results Sheet is used to examine a child's borderline or below-cutoff scores across questionnaire age intervals. (*Note:* In 2004, cutoff scores for the 6, 10, 14, 18, 22, 27, 33, 42, and 54 month intervals were revised. The revised cutoffs for these intervals appear in this figure and in the fifth and subsequent printings of the English and Spanish ASQ questionnaires and also apply to the French ASQ. The revised cutoffs are also posted on-line at http://www.brookespublishing.com/asqupdates/)

Figure 21. *(continued)*

Date completed ______________________

10 months	Score	Cutoff
Communication		25.0
Gross motor		17.5
Fine motor		39.0
Problem solving		30.5
Personal-social		30.0

Communication / Gross motor / Fine motor / Problem solving / Personal-social: items 1–6, Y S N

Comments:

Date completed ______________________

12 months/1 year	Score	Cutoff
Communication		15.8
Gross motor		18.0
Fine motor		28.4
Problem solving		25.2
Personal-social		20.1

Communication / Gross motor / Fine motor / Problem solving / Personal-social: items 1–6, Y S N

Comments:

Date completed ______________________

14 months	Score	Cutoff
Communication		31.0
Gross motor		24.0
Fine motor		25.0
Problem solving		28.5
Personal-social		22.5

Communication / Gross motor / Fine motor / Problem solving / Personal-social: items 1–6, Y S N

Comments:

Date completed ______________________

16 months	Score	Cutoff
Communication		34.5
Gross motor		32.3
Fine motor		30.6
Problem solving		26.9
Personal-social		26.7

Communication / Gross motor / Fine motor / Problem solving / Personal-social: items 1–6, Y S N

Comments:

(continued)

Figure 21. *(continued)*

Date completed ____________________

18 months	Score	Cutoff
Communication		**23.0**
Gross motor		**41.5**
Fine motor		**39.5**
Problem solving		**33.0**
Personal-social		**37.0**

	Communication			Gross motor			Fine motor			Problem solving			Personal-social		
	Y	S	N	Y	S	N	Y	S	N	Y	S	N	Y	S	N
1															
2															
3															
4															
5															
6															

Comments:

Date completed ____________________

20 months	Score	Cutoff
Communication		**36.3**
Gross motor		**36.2**
Fine motor		**39.8**
Problem solving		**29.9**
Personal-social		**35.2**

	Communication			Gross motor			Fine motor			Problem solving			Personal-social		
	Y	S	N	Y	S	N	Y	S	N	Y	S	N	Y	S	N
1															
2															
3															
4															
5															
6															

Comments:

Date completed ____________________

22 months	Score	Cutoff
Communication		**35.0**
Gross motor		**40.0**
Fine motor		**36.5**
Problem solving		**36.5**
Personal-social		**39.5**

	Communication			Gross motor			Fine motor			Problem solving			Personal-social		
	Y	S	N	Y	S	N	Y	S	N	Y	S	N	Y	S	N
1															
2															
3															
4															
5															
6															

Comments:

Date completed ____________________

24 months/2 years	Score	Cutoff
Communication		**36.5**
Gross motor		**36.0**
Fine motor		**36.4**
Problem solving		**32.9**
Personal-social		**35.6**

	Communication			Gross motor			Fine motor			Problem solving			Personal-social		
	Y	S	N	Y	S	N	Y	S	N	Y	S	N	Y	S	N
1															
2															
3															
4															
5															
6															

Comments:

(continued)

Figure 21. *(continued)*

Date completed ______________________

27 months	Score	Cutoff
Communication		**33.5**
Gross motor		**35.0**
Fine motor		**26.0**
Problem solving		**37.0**
Personal-social		**33.0**

	Communication	Gross motor	Fine motor	Problem solving	Personal-social
1					
2					
3					
4					
5					
6					
	Y S N	Y S N	Y S N	Y S N	Y S N

Comments:

Date completed ______________________

30 months	Score	Cutoff
Communication		**38.8**
Gross motor		**30.6**
Fine motor		**25.2**
Problem solving		**28.9**
Personal-social		**36.9**

	Communication	Gross motor	Fine motor	Problem solving	Personal-social
1					
2					
3					
4					
5					
6					
	Y S N	Y S N	Y S N	Y S N	Y S N

Comments:

Date completed ______________________

33 months	Score	Cutoff
Communication		**35.0**
Gross motor		**41.5**
Fine motor		**29.0**
Problem solving		**36.5**
Personal-social		**36.0**

	Communication	Gross motor	Fine motor	Problem solving	Personal-social
1					
2					
3					
4					
5					
6					
	Y S N	Y S N	Y S N	Y S N	Y S N

Comments:

Date completed ______________________

36 months/3 years	Score	Cutoff
Communication		**38.7**
Gross motor		**35.7**
Fine motor		**30.7**
Problem solving		**38.6**
Personal-social		**38.7**

	Communication	Gross motor	Fine motor	Problem solving	Personal-social
1					
2					
3					
4					
5					
6					
	Y S N	Y S N	Y S N	Y S N	Y S N

Comments:

(continued)

Figure 21. *(continued)*

Date completed ______________________

42 months	Score	Cutoff
Communication		38.0
Gross motor		45.0
Fine motor		40.0
Problem solving		39.0
Personal-social		42.5

	Communication			Gross motor			Fine motor			Problem solving			Personal-social		
	Y	S	N	Y	S	N	Y	S	N	Y	S	N	Y	S	N
1	○	○	○	○	○	○	○	○	○	○	○	○	○	○	○
2	○	○	○	○	○	○	○	○	○	○	○	○	○	○	○
3	○	○	○	○	○	○	○	○	○	○	○	○	○	○	○
4	○	○	○	○	○	○	○	○	○	○	○	○	○	○	○
5	○	○	○	○	○	○	○	○	○	○	○	○	○	○	○
6	○	○	○	○	○	○	○	○	○	○	○	○	○	○	○

Comments:

Date completed ______________________

48 months/4 years	Score	Cutoff
Communication		39.1
Gross motor		32.9
Fine motor		30.0
Problem solving		35.0
Personal-social		23.4

	Communication			Gross motor			Fine motor			Problem solving			Personal-social		
	Y	S	N	Y	S	N	Y	S	N	Y	S	N	Y	S	N
1	○	○	○	○	○	○	○	○	○	○	○	○	○	○	○
2	○	○	○	○	○	○	○	○	○	○	○	○	○	○	○
3	○	○	○	○	○	○	○	○	○	○	○	○	○	○	○
4	○	○	○	○	○	○	○	○	○	○	○	○	○	○	○
5	○	○	○	○	○	○	○	○	○	○	○	○	○	○	○
6	○	○	○	○	○	○	○	○	○	○	○	○	○	○	○

Comments:

Date completed ______________________

54 months	Score	Cutoff
Communication		50.0
Gross motor		42.5
Fine motor		26.5
Problem solving		33.0
Personal-social		36.5

	Communication			Gross motor			Fine motor			Problem solving			Personal-social		
	Y	S	N	Y	S	N	Y	S	N	Y	S	N	Y	S	N
1	○	○	○	○	○	○	○	○	○	○	○	○	○	○	○
2	○	○	○	○	○	○	○	○	○	○	○	○	○	○	○
3	○	○	○	○	○	○	○	○	○	○	○	○	○	○	○
4	○	○	○	○	○	○	○	○	○	○	○	○	○	○	○
5	○	○	○	○	○	○	○	○	○	○	○	○	○	○	○
6	○	○	○	○	○	○	○	○	○	○	○	○	○	○	○

Comments:

Date completed ______________________

60 months/5 years	Score	Cutoff
Communication		31.7
Gross motor		32.7
Fine motor		30.5
Problem solving		30.1
Personal-social		39.5

	Communication			Gross motor			Fine motor			Problem solving			Personal-social		
	Y	S	N	Y	S	N	Y	S	N	Y	S	N	Y	S	N
1	○	○	○	○	○	○	○	○	○	○	○	○	○	○	○
2	○	○	○	○	○	○	○	○	○	○	○	○	○	○	○
3	○	○	○	○	○	○	○	○	○	○	○	○	○	○	○
4	○	○	○	○	○	○	○	○	○	○	○	○	○	○	○
5	○	○	○	○	○	○	○	○	○	○	○	○	○	○	○
6	○	○	○	○	○	○	○	○	○	○	○	○	○	○	○

Comments:

vals. Interpreting ASQ scores is also discussed in the videotape *ASQ Scoring & Referral.* ***In all instances, it is important not to alarm parents but to emphasize that the score indicates only that further evaluation or follow-up is in order.*** The recommended procedures for children whose questionnaire scores meet the referral criteria are as follows:

1. Call or visit the parents. Explain that the questionnaire identified some concerns about their child's development and that further testing is recommended. Suggestions for talking to parents about ASQ scores are provided in Table 5. Ask parents to talk about any concerns they may have and request permission to contact the child's primary health care provider by asking parents to sign a release of information.
2. If permission is granted, either contact the child's physician and summarize the questionnaire results or send a letter such as the sample shown in Figure 22.
3. If requested by the parents or physician, arrange for further developmental assessment by providing a referral to an agency that provides developmental testing. The local early intervention council, school district, or health department may be able to provide information about resources for further testing.
4. If appropriate, provide feedback to parents and the physician about the outcome of the developmental assessment.
5. Enter the results of the developmental assessment in the child's file.
6. If the child is found eligible for services and if program resources permit, assist the parents in contacting intervention programs. If the child is not found eligible for intervention services, arrange for completion of the next *Ages & Stages Questionnaire* when the child reaches the appropriate age interval.

To assist in making appropriate and timely referrals, it is helpful to keep up-to-date lists of community agencies that provide developmental assessments and programs that provide intervention services to infants and young children. The list should include the following information for each entry:

- Agency name and address
- Contact person
- Telephone number
- Eligibility criteria for evaluation and/or intervention
- Services provided

Table 5. Suggestions for talking to parents about ASQ results that identify a child for further assessment

- Provide screening information as quickly as possible.
- Use the family's primary language, communicating in clear, simple terms.
- Emphasize that results from a screening tool can be inaccurate and do not provide in-depth information about the child's abilities.
- Avoid judging cultural and linguistic differences or customs.
- Explain the child's score in relation to the ASQ cutoff points.
- Avoid using terms like "fail," "pass," "normal," "abnormal," and "test."
- Emphasize the child's current skills.
- Emphasize the family's current skills and resources.
- Take time to talk about the family's *perception* of their child's resources and areas of concern.
- Talk to the family about additional community services they may obtain.

Dear [fill in physician's name]:

After reviewing and scoring the *Ages & Stages Questionnaire* completed by [fill in parent's name] on your patient, [fill in child's name], we have some concerns about the developmental progress of this child.

We have informed the parents that their child would likely benefit from further developmental assessment, and they have indicated they will make an appointment with you. Please contact us if you have any questions.

Sincerely,

[fill in staff member's name]
[fill in program name]

Figure 22. A sample feedback letter to the physician of a child whose questionnaire scores suggest a developmental delay.

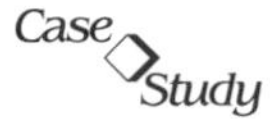

Kinko is 30 months old. Kinko's mother, Choi-yu, has received the *Ages & Stages Questionnaires* by mail for 2½ years. On the 30 month ASQ, Kinko's scores indicate that she is well above the cutoff points and is developing typically. Choi-yu did not indicate any concerns about Kinko's development in the Overall section. Kinko originally was referred to Steps-Ahead because she was born 6 weeks prematurely and because Choi-yu was being treated for chronic depression. Steps-Ahead sent Choi-yu a copy of the completed 30 month ASQ, the Intervention Activities Sheet for 30 months, and a letter similar to the one shown in Figure 20. Steps-Ahead will continue to monitor Kinko's development and send another questionnaire when she is 33 months old.

Jake is 12 months old. His mother, Naomi, completed the 12 month ASQ in her home with the assistance of a social worker from Steps-Ahead. Jake was referred to Steps-Ahead because his birth weight was extremely low and because Naomi was a teenager with a reported history of substance abuse and domestic violence. Jake's scores on the 12 month ASQ were just above the cutoff points for most areas of development and were below the cutoff point for problem solving. Jake's 8 month ASQ scores were also low but did not fall below the cutoff points. On the Overall section, Naomi indicated that she felt very stressed and was having trouble with Jake's newfound mobility. The Steps-Ahead social worker discussed the results of the questionnaire with Naomi, and a referral for further developmental testing was made. Naomi was linked with agencies that would help provide parenting support. She was given the completed ASQ, and the social worker kept the Information Summary Sheet for Steps-Ahead. After modeling some activities, the social worker also gave Naomi an Intervention Activities Sheet for 12-month-olds. Naomi signed a release to notify Jake's pediatrician of the questionnaire results and Steps-Ahead's recommendation for further testing. Jake was tested

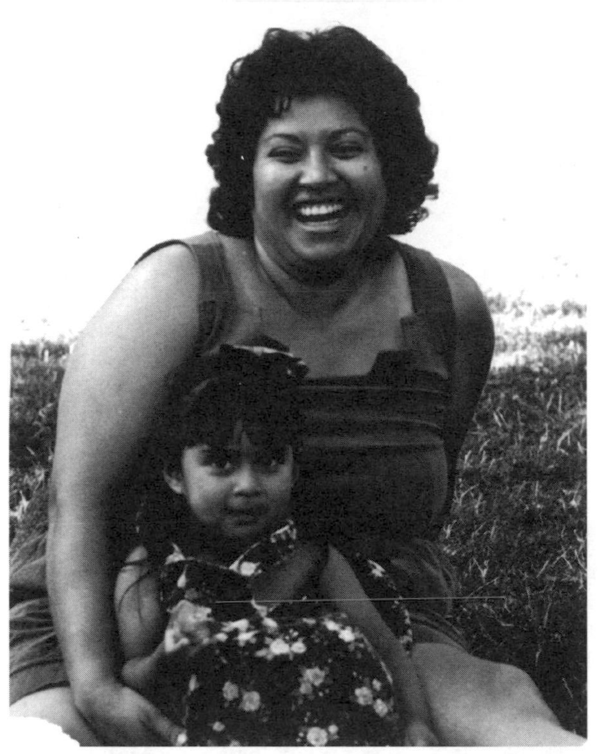

by the early intervention services agency and was found to be eligible for services. Jake will no longer be monitored by Steps-Ahead. His records will be forwarded to the early intervention program after Naomi signs a release form.

Gabriella is 16 months old. Sylvia and Juan, Gabriella's parents, completed the 16 month ASQ in their home with the assistance of a social worker from Steps-Ahead. Gabriella was referred to Steps-Ahead because of her pediatrician's concern about her development and history of chronic ear infections. Gabriella's scores on the questionnaire were well above the cutoff points, except for the communication and problem solving areas, for which her scores were low or near the cutoff points. Gabriella's parents expressed concern in the Overall section in response to the question, "Do you think your child talks like other toddlers his (or her) age?" Earlier, Gabriella's parents completed questionnaires when she was 8 and 12 months old. Both of these questionnaires showed Gabriella's development to be well above the cutoff points in all areas. Given the results of Gabriella's 16 month questionnaire and the noted parental concerns, the Steps-Ahead social worker called her parents to discuss options. Sylvia and Juan decided to wait and watch Gabriella's development in the communication and problem-solving areas. The social worker gave Sylvia and Juan the 16 month questionnaire and an Intervention Activities Sheet for 16 months. The social worker also gave Gabriella's parents the 20 month questionnaire and the corresponding Intervention Activities Sheet to help them watch for skills that Gabriella should begin to develop in the coming months. Steps-Ahead will continue to monitor Gabriella's development with the *Ages & Stages Questionnaires.* Special attention will be given to the communication and problem solving areas on the 20 month ASQ.

Jeffery is 20 months old. He lives with his grandmother and his brother and sister. Jeffery's grandmother completes the questionnaires, which she receives by mail. Jeffery was referred to Steps-Ahead because he was prenatally exposed to drugs and had a history of abuse by his biological mother. Jeffery's grandmother has completed questionnaires since he was 8 months old. Results from these questionnaires indicate that Jeffery's development is well above the cutoff points; however, his grandmother has noted that Jeffery is unable to sleep at night. She reported that she finds him in their living room in the morning, asleep on the couch. The Steps-Ahead social worker called Jeffery's grandmother to discuss her concerns. Based on their discussion, the social worker recommended that Jeffery be seen by his pediatrician to evaluate his sleeping problem. In the meantime, the social worker returned to Jeffery's grandmother the completed 20 month ASQ and the Intervention Activities Sheet for that age interval. Upon examination, Jeffery's pediatrician found that he had asthma and prescribed appropriate medication. Jeffery's grandmother reported to Steps-Ahead that Jeffery's sleeping habits have improved. Steps-Ahead will continue to monitor Jeffery's development with the *Ages & Stages Questionnaires.*

CONCLUSION

Phase II, using and scoring the questionnaires, contains the steps necessary for the daily operations of the monitoring system. The first step, assembling the child file, ensures that all questionnaires and forms will be kept in a single location and can be easily found. Step 2, keeping track of the questionnaires, pertains to establishing an efficient system for mailing or presenting the questionnaires to families within the target date "window." Step 3, using the questionnaires, details the various ways in which questionnaires can be presented to families. Procedures for mail-out, one-time screening, telephone interviews, home visits, and use in primary care medical offices are described. The fourth step, scoring the questionnaires, provides instructions for scoring and recording results of the ASQ. Although the scoring instructions may seem complicated on the first reading, a short practice session with two or three questionnaires will clarify most concerns. Step 5, determining follow-up, reviews suggestions for giving feedback to parents whose children score above the cutoff points, indicating typical development. In addition, suggestions are reviewed for talking to parents about possible referral for further evaluation of children whose questionnaire scores fall below the cutoff points and/or when parental concerns are noted in the Overall section.

This *User's Guide* is intended to be a reference; there are many sections in this chapter that will need to be reviewed as monitoring program operations begin. Options such as those for using questionnaires and ways to give parents feedback may need to be tried until a system that fits individual program needs is established. Chapter 6 describes the final phase of the ASQ system, evaluating the monitoring program.

6

Phase III: Evaluating the Monitoring Program

ASQ™

Phase III of the ASQ system focuses on evaluating the monitoring program in terms of both the program's implementation progress and the effectiveness of the screening tool. This phase has two steps, which are shown in the shaded portion of Figure 23. As with any system, each step in the ASQ system should lead to the next. As indicated in Figure 23, the evaluation of the ASQ system provides information about the attainment of program goals and may simultaneously suggest new goals. Ongoing evaluation may result in the modification of procedures and steps in all three phases of the program.

Contemplating the evaluation of the screening process should not begin at the end of Phase II. Rather, knowing the goals of the evaluation process facilitates collecting information needed as the program progresses.

STEPS IN PHASE III: EVALUATING THE MONITORING PROGRAM

Assess Progress in the Establishment and Maintenance of the Monitoring Program

Setting up and maintaining a screening and monitoring program for a large number of children require a range of activities. The Implementation Progress Worksheet shown in Figure 24 was developed to assist program personnel in efficiently monitoring the variety of required phases and steps necessary for initiation and maintenance of the program. The items on this worksheet mirror the 14 steps in the three phases of the ASQ system. The worksheet is intended to be of assistance during the initiation and early stages of developing the monitoring program; however, staff may find it useful to refer back to the worksheet at designated intervals (e.g., quarterly) even after the program has been institutionalized.

The left column of the Implementation Progress Worksheet lists each of the 14 steps in the ASQ process (e.g., establish goals and objectives, determine program resources) in the order they are described in this *User's Guide.* To the right of this column are five "action" columns: personnel needs, information needs, supplies and equipment needs, person/agency responsible, and projected date of completion. Personnel can enter in each column the indicated information for the individual steps.

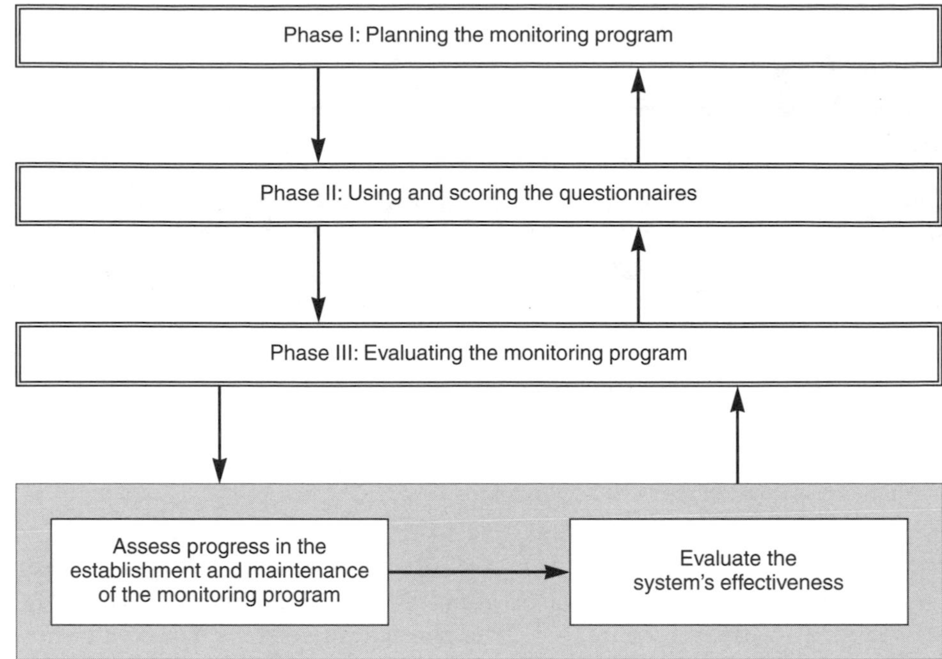

Figure 23. The two steps in Phase III of the ASQ system are in the shaded area. Their crucial connection to the earlier phases is illustrated as well. The data collected from these evaluation steps permit constant improvement of the system.

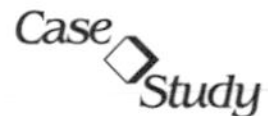

For the Involve Parents step, personnel from the Steps-Ahead program might enter the following information:

Personnel Needs: *Social workers* to make individual contacts with parents of infants identified on birth certificates and *clerical staff* to type letters to parents and to take telephone messages

Information Needs: Current names, addresses, and telephone numbers (if available) of families

Supplies and Equipment Needs: Secretarial supplies, including *stamps, computer and software for word processing, letterhead, and a telephone with two lines*

Person/Agency Responsible: *Social workers* will have responsibil-ity for *obtaining consent to participate from parents;* thereafter, *social workers* will have responsibility for *ongoing contact with participating parents* and for *altering the ASQ method of use when requested*

Projected Date of Completion: Parents to be contacted for consent *within 1 month after birth of child or within 1 month after child returns home from the hospital*

The final column provides four spaces to indicate the quantitative level of progress attained toward the specific step's completion. The rating scale includes the following numerical values:

Implementation Progress Worksheet

Tasks	Actions					Progress rating			
	Personnel needs	Information needs	Supplies and equipment needs	Person/ agency responsible	Projected date of completion				
Phase I: Planning the monitoring program									
1 Establish goals and objectives									
2 Determine program resources									
3 Determine method of use									
4 Select criteria for participation in the program									
5 Involve parents									
6 Involve physicians									
7 Outline referral criteria									

(continued)

Figure 24. The Implementation Progress Worksheet can be used by program personnel to monitor the phases and steps in the initiation and maintenance of a program administering the *Ages & Stages Questionnaires.* For progress ratings: 0 = Not applicable; 1 = Not begun; 2 = Partially begun or implemented; 3 = Fully completed or implemented.

Figure 24. *(continued)*

Implementation Progress Worksheet

Tasks	Actions					Progress rating			
	Personnel needs	Information needs	Supplies and equipment needs	Person/ agency responsible	Projected date of completion				
Phase II: Using and scoring the questionnaires									
8 Assemble the child file									
9 Keep track of the questionnaires									
10 Use the questionnaires									
11 Score the questionnaires									
12 Determine follow-up									

Figure 24. *(continued)*

Tasks	Actions					Progress rating			
	Personnel needs	Information needs	Supplies and equipment needs	Person/ agency responsible	Projected date of completion				
Phase III: Evaluating the monitoring program									
13 Assess progress in establishing and maintaining the program									
14 Evaluate effectiveness									

(continued)

Figure 24. *(continued)*

Implementation Progress Worksheet

Additional Program Needs

1. ______________________________
2. ______________________________
3. ______________________________
4. ______________________________
5. ______________________________

Summary: ______________________________

0 = Not applicable
1 = Not begun
2 = Partially begun or implemented
3 = Fully completed or implemented

During initial start-up, program staff may want to evaluate their progress weekly using the Implementation Progress Worksheet. Later, monthly or quarterly evaluations of progress may be sufficient. Tasks to evaluate will change as the program matures and as more children are being monitored. As program objectives are modified, it may be necessary to begin a new worksheet reflecting these new objectives.

For example, for Step 5, Involve Parents, analyzed in the case study in Chapter 4, the goal of garnering parents' support of the monitoring program 1 month after the birth of their child may be too soon. This task may need to be changed to contacting and mailing information to parents at 1 month and waiting until the infant is 2 months or older to make a home visit and explain the ASQ system.

Although most programs will strive for ratings of 3 on targeted steps, there may be instances in which a rating of 2 is sufficient. Limited resources, lower priority, or modification of steps may be reasons for these lower ratings. If a modification occurs, steps should be rewritten and reevaluated.

Evaluate the System's Effectiveness

The final step shown in Figure 23 is Evaluate the System's Effectiveness. Every monitoring program, even those with limited resources, should conduct some form of evaluation to determine the effectiveness of the program and the procedures being used. The following areas of evaluation are recommended:

- Parent feedback
- Effectiveness of questionnaires in accurately identifying children in need of further assessment
- Feedback from personnel using the questionnaires
- Simple analyses of sensitivity, specificity, overreferral, underreferral, and percent of children identified for further assessment (Appendix F addresses each of these areas.)

How extensively each of these areas can be evaluated will depend on the program's resources and staff expertise. The evaluation procedures described next are simple and straightforward; they represent the minimal amount of evaluation each program should conduct.

Feedback from parents should be sought at least yearly. A simple, short survey can be devised and included with a questionnaire once a year (e.g., 12, 24, 36, 48, 60 months). Figure 25 is an example of such a survey.

To examine the effectiveness of the questionnaires, it is imperative to keep records of the number of children identified as needing further assessment and the outcome of their subsequent developmental assessments. By recording this information, it is possible to determine the percent of children accurately identified by the questionnaires as having delays and those who were incorrectly recommended for further evaluation. These calculations provide information on the sensitivity and overreferral rates for the group of children being monitored. Providing information on the effectiveness of a screening program may help personnel in a variety of ways. First, data on the

Dear Parent,

Would you please take a few minutes to evaluate our questionnaires? We appreciate your participation in our program and hope that our services have been helpful to you.

Please circle the number that best expresses your opinion.

1. Approximately how many minutes did it take you to fill out each questionnaire? ______ minutes
   Did you consider this amount of time:

very little time			too much time
1	2	3	4

Comments:

2. Did the questionnaires alert you to skills or activities your child could do that you were not sure about?

very few			very many
1	2	3	4

Comments:

3. After filling out the questionnaires, did you have any new ideas about how to interact or play with your child?

very few			very many
1	2	3	4

Comments:

4. Were any items unclear or difficult to understand?

very few			very many
1	2	3	4

Comments:

5. Did you enjoy participating in this program?

very little			very much
1	2	3	4

Comments:

If you have any further comments about the questionnaires, please write them on the back of this form.

Figure 25. An example of a feedback form sent to parents participating in the program. Such a survey should be distributed at least once a year, if possible. A Spanish translation of this form is provided in Appendix C.

effectiveness of the screening program may be requested and appreciated by funding sources. Second, additional information may be provided about the monitoring of implementation goals. For example, a program may project a screening rate of 10%. By calculating the percentage of children identified, the percent identified is obtained. If the program's goal of 10% is not realized (i.e., percent screened is significantly higher or lower), the criteria used to include children in the program may need to be modified.

		Follow-up assessment	
		Intervention needs	No intervention needs
Ages & Stages Questionnaires	Identified by questionnaires as needing further assessment	True positives A	False positives (overreferral) B
	Not identified by questionnaires; developing typically	False negatives (underreferral) C	True negatives D

Percent of children identified as needing further assessment:

$$\frac{A + B}{A + B + C + D}$$

Sensitivity The proportion of children correctly identified by the questionnaires as needing further assessment:

$$\frac{A}{A + C}$$

Specificity The proportion of children correctly identified by the questionnaires as developing typically:

$$\frac{D}{B + D}$$

Overreferral The proportion of children (of the total number of children for whom a questionnaire was completed) incorrectly identified by the questionnaires as needing further assessment:

$$\frac{B}{A + B + C + D}$$

Underreferral The proportion of children (of the total number of children for whom a questionnaire was completed) incorrectly excluded by the questionnaires:

$$\frac{C}{A + B + C + D}$$

Positive predictive value The proportion of children identified by the questionnaires as needing further assessment who will, in fact, have intervention needs:

$$\frac{A}{A + B}$$

Figure 26. Contingency table, definitions, and formulas for evaluating the effectiveness of the ASQ monitoring program.

Figure 26 provides formulas for calculating the percent of children appropriately identified as needing further assessment, as well as the sensitivity, specificity, and overreferral and underreferral rates.[1]

Finally, it is important to seek formal or informal feedback from personnel using the questionnaires, learning from them which program proce-

[1]Specificity and underreferral rates cannot be calculated unless a program conducts follow-up assessments with children who are not identified by the questionnaires as needing further assessment, as well as with children identified as needing further assessment.

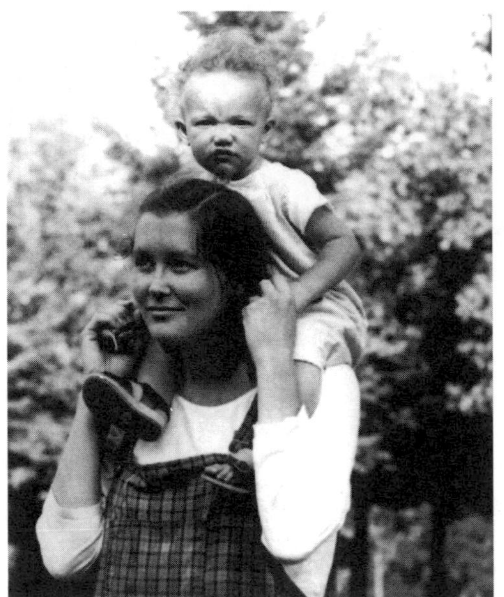

dures work well and which ones do not. The ASQ system is flexible, and program personnel can and should make adjustments in its use to ensure efficient and effective application. At least once a year, staff should meet to examine ways to improve the activities associated with their monitoring program.

Case Study

After 6 months, the Steps-Ahead staff reviewed their progress in completing targeted tasks (Figure 27). For the planning phase, goals and objectives, program resources, and method of use steps were fully implemented and had met projected dates of completion. Criteria for participation, involving parents and physicians, and determining referral criteria were only partially implemented, receiving ratings of 2. Although criteria for participation and for referral had been determined, it was believed that more time was needed to evaluate how these guidelines were functioning within program parameters. Staff decided to continue to record the numbers of children served and numbers of children referred for further evaluation; in 3 months the staff would meet to evaluate how well these actual numbers corresponded with their projections.

In terms of involving physicians, more work was needed to inform physicians at private hospitals in the area and to garner support from the health maintenance organizations at these private hospitals. Advisory board staff, as well as social workers, were designated to work with the private hospitals.

In terms of involving parents, staff felt positive about their relationships with families. However, they decided to add two parents to the advisory board so that parent input would be ongoing. Staff also undertook the development of a satisfaction questionnaire for parents to complete along with the 12 month questionnaire.

Regarding Phase II, using and scoring the questionnaires, all clerical and office tasks related to setting up and maintaining child files had been completed. Procedures for the tickler system, scoring, and recording questionnaire results appeared to be working well. For these clerical and office tasks, staff decided to reevaluate progress in 3 months, when there were larger numbers of children participating in the monitoring system.

For the task of determining follow-up for children who are identified as needing further assessment, staff believed that, to date, there were insufficient numbers to rate progress. The early intervention program in the county had evaluated 6 of the 10 children referred to date and had shared results with Steps-Ahead. Parents of two of the identified children had requested further monitoring with the questionnaires before referral. Two children had been evaluated by physicians at a health maintenance organization, but these results had not been received by Steps-Ahead.

Implementation Progress Worksheet

Tasks	Actions					Progress rating			
	Personnel needs	Information needs	Supplies and equipment needs	Person/ agency responsible	Projected date of completion				
Phase I: Planning the monitoring program						*3/1*	*6/1*		
1 Establish goals and objectives	*Schedule three 2-hour staff meetings to discuss, outline*	*State and federal regulations*	*Large writing paper and pens*	*Director*	*12/1*	*3*			
2 Determine program resources	*Social workers, advisory board; Director*	*Available resources and in-kind contributions*	*Computer software for word processor, database*	*Director*	*1/1*	*3*			
3 Determine method of use	*Staff, advisory board*	*Available resources (#2), needs and characteristics of parents*	*Copy machine, box and file cards for tickler system*	*Director*	*2/1*	*3*			
4 Select criteria for participation in the program	*Physicians, nurses on advisory board; 2 meetings*	*Risk criteria from research studies*	*Library, computer search capabilities*	*Director to assist with search and schedule meetings*	*1/1*	*2*			
5 Involve parents	*Social workers—contact parents; clerical staff—letters, telephone*	*Names, addresses, telephone numbers*	*Secretarial supplies, telephone, computer, software*	*Social workers*	*Parent contact 1 month after birth*	*2*			
6 Involve physicians	*Physicians, nurses on advisory board*	*Names of physicians at HMOs, medical society lists*	*Mailing labels, telephone, word processor*	*Advisory board—physician contacts, clerical staff—letters*	*2/1*	*2*			
7 Outline referral criteria	*Advisory board, social workers*	*List of community resources for evaluation, cutoffs from User's Guide*	*Word processor*	*Directors*	*2/1*	*2*			

(continued)

Figure 27. The staff at Steps-Ahead completed an Implementation Progress Worksheet to monitor their progress. Their status at 6 months is shown here.

Figure 27. *(continued)*

Implementation Progress Worksheet

Tasks	Actions					Progress rating			
	Personnel needs	Information needs	Supplies and equipment needs	Person/ agency responsible	Projected date of completion				
Phase II: Using and scoring the questionnaires						*3/1*	*6/1*		
8 Assemble the child file	*Clerical staff*	*ID # system, family information*	*File folders, labels*	*Clerical staff*	*2/1*	*3*			
9 Keep track of the questionnaires	*Social workers*	*Child's date of birth and family information*	*Tickler system— file boxes, cards, dividers*	*Social workers*	*2/1*	*3*			
10 Use the questionnaires	*Social workers*	*Directions from User's Guide*	*ASQ at each interval, letters from User's Guide*	*Social workers*	*2/1*	*3*			
11 Score the questionnaires	*Social workers*	*Scoring directions from User's Guide*	*Information Summary Sheets from ASQ*	*Social workers*	*2/1*	*3*			
12 Determine follow-up	*Social workers*	*Referral criteria (#7), availability of community evaluation and support services*	*List of community resources, telephone numbers*	*Social workers— contacts with referral sources, Director— contacts with physicians*	*3/1*	*2 reevaluate*			

Figure 27. *(continued)*

Implementation Progress Worksheet

Tasks	Actions					Progress rating			
	Personnel needs	Information needs	Supplies and equipment needs	Person/ agency responsible	Projected date of completion				
Phase III: Evaluating the Monitoring Program						*3/1*	*6/1*		
13 Assess progress in establishing and maintaining the program	*Monthly staff meetings*	*Progress worksheet*	*Clerical supplies, computer*	*Director*	*3/1—Evaluate overall progress*	2			
14 Evaluate effectiveness	*Social workers, Director*	*Outcomes from child evaluations, public school placements for 4- to 5-year-olds*	*Computer, calculator, formulas from User's Guide*	*Director*	*3/1*	2			

(continued)

Figure 27. *(continued)*

Implementation Progress Worksheet

Additional Program Needs

1. *Ensure links between Steps-Ahead and early intervention programs so that Steps-Ahead can find out what the outcomes are for children referred for assessment.*
2. *Identify and ask two parents to join the advisory board.*
3. *Develop and circulate parent satisfaction questionnaire.*
4. __________
5. __________

Summary: __________

For Phase III, evaluating the monitoring program, the Implementation Progress Worksheet had been completed and all steps had been rated (see Figure 27). Steps receiving ratings of 2 were targeted, and staff had been assigned new tasks. Progress toward full implementation of these steps was to be evaluated during monthly staff meetings. The next program evaluation meeting was scheduled for 3 months later.

CONCLUSION

Phase III, evaluating the monitoring program, involves two steps—assessing progress in the establishment and maintenance of the monitoring program and evaluating the system's effectiveness. Progress can be assessed by monitoring project staff during monthly or quarterly staff meetings and should not require extensive information or data that go beyond day-to-day operations of the program. The second step, evaluating the system's effectiveness, is also of prime importance. Information may be needed from outside referral agencies to determine child evaluation outcomes. These data are necessary in order to determine whether the program is really working: Are the right children being identified for further evaluation? Are they then referred for early intervention services? Evaluation of the monitoring program should be ongoing, and revision of steps and activities will be necessary as the program grows and changes.

References

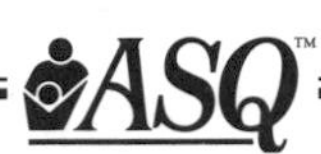

Bayley, N. (1969). *Bayley Scales of Infant Development.* San Antonio, TX: The Psychological Corp.

Behrman, R.E. (Ed.). (1997). The future of children. *Children and poverty, (7)*2.

Benn, R. (1993). Conceptualizing eligibility for services. In D. Bryant & M. Grahm (Eds.), *Implementing early intervention* (pp. 18–45). New York: Guilford Press.

Bricker, D., & Squires, J. (1989). Low cost system using parents to monitor the development of at risk infants. *Journal of Early Intervention, 13,* 50–60.

Bricker, D., Squires, J., Kaminski, R., & Mounts, L. (1988). The validity, reliability, and cost of a parent-completed questionnaire system to evaluate at-risk infants. *Journal of Pediatric Psychology, 13*(1), 56–68.

Chan, B., & Taylor, N. (1998). The follow-along program cost analysis in southwest Minnesota. *Infants and Young Children, 10*(4), 71–79.

Clark, R., Paulson, A., & Conlin, S. (1993). Assessment of developmental status and parent–infant relationships: The therapeutic process of evaluation. In C. Zeanah (Ed.), *Handbook of infant mental health* (pp. 191–209). New York: Guilford Press.

Davidson, J., & Cripe, J. (1987). *Intervention activities.* Eugene: University of Oregon Infant Monitoring Project.

Education of the Handicapped Act Amendments of 1983, PL 98-199, 20 U.S.C. §§ 1400 *et seq.*

Education of the Handicapped Act Amendments of 1986, PL 99-457, 20 U.S.C. §§ 1400 *et seq.*

Farrell, J., & Potter, L. (Developers). (1995). *The Ages & Stages Questionnaires on a home visit* [Videotape]. Baltimore: Paul H. Brookes Publishing Co.

Frankenburg, W.K., & Dodds, J.B. (1970). *Denver Developmental Screening Test (DDST).* Denver, CO: Ladoca Project and Publishing Foundation, Inc.

Frankenburg, W., Van Doorninck, W., Liddell, T., & Dick, N. (1976). The Denver Prescreening Developmental Questionnaire (PDQ). *Pediatrics, 57,* 744–753.

Individuals with Disabilities Education Act (IDEA) of 1990, PL 101-476, 20 U.S.C. §§ 1400 *et seq.*

Individuals with Disabilities Education Act Amendments of 1997, PL 105-17, 20 U.S.C. §§ 1400 *et seq.*

Knobloch, H., Stevens, F., & Malone, A.F. (1980). *Manual of developmental diagnosis: The administration and interpretation of the Revised Gesell and Amatruda Developmental and Neurological Examination.* New York: Harper & Row.

Knobloch, H., Stevens, F., Malone, A., Ellison, P., & Risemburg, H. (1979). The validity of parental reporting of infant development. *Pediatrics, 63,* 873–878.

Mardell-Czudnowski, C., & Goldenberg, D. (1983). *Developmental Indicators for the Assessment of Learning–Revised (DIAL–R).* Edison, NJ: Childcraft Education.

McCarthy, D. (1972). *McCarthy Scales of Children's Abilities.* San Antonio, TX: The Psychological Corp.

Meisels, S., & Provence, S. (1989). *Screening and assessment: Guidelines for identifying young disabled and developmentally vulnerable children and their families.* Washington, DC: National Center for Clinical Infant Programs.

Meisels, S., & Wiske, M. (1982). *Early Screening Inventory.* New York: Teachers College Press.

Mitchell, S., Bee, H., Hammond, M., & Barnard, K. (1985). Prediction of school and behavior problems in children followed from birth to age eight. In W. Frankenburg, R. Emde, & J. Sullivan (Eds.), *Early identification of children at risk* (pp. 117–132). New York: Plenum.

Newborg, J., Stock, J.R., Wnek, L., Guidubaldi, J., & Svinicki, J. (1987). *Battelle Developmental Inventory.* Chicago: Riverside.

Sameroff, A., Seifer, R., Barocas, B., Zax, M., & Greenspan, S. (1987). IQ scores of 4-year-old children: Socio-environmental risk factors. *Pediatrics, 79*(3), 343–350.

Squires, J., & Bricker, D. (1991). Impact of completing infant developmental questionnaires on at-risk mothers. *Journal of Early Intervention, 15*(2), 162–172.

Squires, J., Bricker, D., & Potter, L. (1997). Revision of a parent-completed developmental screening tool: Ages and Stages Questionnaires. *Journal of Pediatric Psychology, 22*(3), 313–328.

Squires, J., Nickel, R., & Bricker, D. (1990). Use of parent-completed developmental questionnaires for Child-Find and screening. *Infants and Young Children, 3*(2), 46–57.

Squires, J., Nickel, R., & Eisert, D. (1996). Early detection of developmental problems: Strategies for monitoring young children in the practice setting. *Journal of Developmental and Behavioral Pediatrics, 17*(6), 410–427.

Thorndike, R., Hagen, E., & Sattler, J. (1985). *Stanford-Binet Intelligence Scale* (4th ed.). Chicago: Riverside.

III APPENDICES

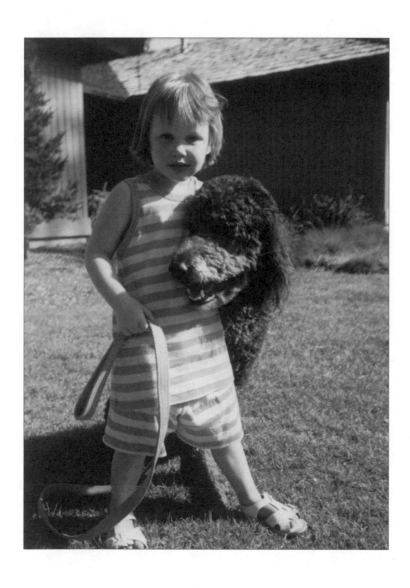

A

Suggested Readings

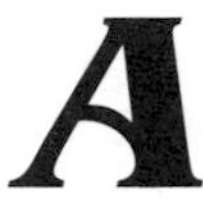

Bennett, F., Nickel, R., Squires, J., & Woodward, B. (1997). Developmental screening/surveillance. In H. Wallace, R. Biehl, R. MacQueen, & J. Blackman (Eds.), *Children with disabilities and chronic illnesses* (pp. 236–247). Oakland, CA: Mosby Yearbook.

Bernbaum, J.C., & Batshaw, M.L. (1997). Born too soon, born too small. In M.L. Batshaw (Ed.), *Children with disabilities* (4th ed., pp. 115–139). Baltimore: Paul H. Brookes Publishing Co.

Blackman, J. (1986). *Warning signals: Basic criteria for tracking at-risk infants and toddlers.* Washington, DC: National Center for Clinical Infant Programs.

Bricker, D., & Littman, D. (1985). Parental monitoring of infant development. In R. McMahon & R. Peters (Eds.), *Childhood disorders: Behavioral-developmental approaches* (pp. 90–115). New York: Brunner/Mazel.

Bricker, D., & Squires, J. (1989a). Low cost system using parents to monitor the development of at-risk infants. *Journal of Early Intervention, 13,* 50–60.

Bricker, D., & Squires, J. (1989b). The effectiveness of parent screening of at-risk infants: The infant monitoring questionnaires. *Topics in Early Childhood Special Education, 9*(3), 67–85.

Bricker, D., Squires, J., Kaminski, R., & Mounts, L. (1988). The validity, reliability, and cost of a parent-completed questionnaire system to evaluate at-risk infants. *Journal of Pediatric Psychology, 13*(1), 56–68.

Chan, B., & Taylor, N. (1998). The follow along program cost analysis in southwest Minnesota. *Infants & Young Children, 10*(4), 71–79.

Committee on Children with Disabilities. (2001, July). Developmental surveillance and screening of infants and young children. *Pediatrics, 108,* 192–196.

Diamond, K., & Squires, J. (1993). The role of parental report in the screening and assessment of young children. *Journal of Early Intervention, 17*(2), 107–115.

Dobrez, D., Sasso, A.L., Holl, J., Shalowitz, M., Leon, S., & Budetti, P. (2001). Estimating the cost of developmental and behavioral screening of preschool children in general pediatric practice. *Pediatrics, 108,* 913–922.

Dworkin, P., & Glascoe, F. (1997). Early detection of developmental delays: How do you measure up? *Contemporary Pediatrics, 14*(4), 158–168.

Filipek, P., Accardo, P., Ashwal, S., Baranek, G.T., Cook, E.H., Jr., Dawson, G., et al. (2000). Practice parameter: screening and diagnosis of autism. A report of the quality standards subcommittee of American Academy of Neurology and the Child Neurology Society. *Neurology, 55,* 468–479.

First, L., & Palfrey, J. (1994). The infant or young child with developmental delay. *New England Journal of Medicine, 330*(7), 478–483.

Glascoe, F. (1991). Developmental screening: Rationale, methods, and application. *Infants and Young Children, 4*(1), 1–10.

Glascoe, F.P. (2000, March). Evidence-based approach to developmental and behavioral surveillance using parents' concerns. *Child: Care, Health & Development, 26*(2), 137–149.

Glascoe, F., Martin, E., & Humphrey, S. (1990). Consumer reports: A comparative review of developmental screening tests. *Pediatrics, 86*(4), 547–553.

Hack, M., Breslau, N., Weissman, B., Aram, D., Klein, N., & Borawski, E. (1991). Effect of very low birth weight and subnormal head size on cognitive abilities at school age. *New England Journal of Medicine, 325*(4), 231–277.

Janson, H. (2003). Influences on participation rate in a national Norwegian child development screening questionnaire study. *Acta Paediatrica, 92*(1), 91–96.

Janson, H., & Squires, J. (2004). Parent-completed developmental screening in a Norwegian population sample: A comparison with U.S. normative data. *Acta Paediatrica, 93,* 1525–1529.

Knobloch, H., Stevens, F., Malone, A.F., Ellison, P., & Risemburg, H. (1979). The validity of parental reporting of infant development. *Pediatrics, 63,* 873–878.

Kochanek, T. (1993). Enhancing screening procedures for infants and toddlers: The application of knowledge to public policy and program initiatives. In D. Bryant & M. Graham (Eds.), *Implementing early intervention: From research to effective practice* (pp. 46–66). New York: Guilford Press.

Lichtenstein, R., & Ireton, H. (1984). *Preschool screening: Identifying young children with developmental and educational problems.* San Francisco: Grune & Stratton.

Liptak, G. (1996). The pediatrician's role in caring for the developmentally disabled child. *Pediatrics in Review, 17*(6), 203–210.

Meisels, S., & Shonkoff, J. (Eds.). (1990). *Handbook of early childhood intervention.* New York: Cambridge University Press.

National Center for Clinical Infant Programs. (no date). *Keeping track: Tracking systems for high risk infants and young children.* Washington, DC: Author.

Sameroff, A. (1981). Longitudinal studies of preterm infants: A review of chapters 17–20. In S. Friedman & M. Sigman (Eds.), *Preterm birth and psychological development* (pp. 387–393). New York: Academic Press.

Scott, K., & Masi, W. (1979). The outcome from and utility of registers of risk. In T. Field, A. Sostek, S. Goldberg, & H. Shuman (Eds.), *Infants born at risk* (pp. 485–496). Jamaica, NY: Spectrum Publications.

Skellern, C.Y., & O'Callaghan, M. (1999, October). Parent-completed questionnaires: An effective screening instrument for developmental delay in follow-up of ex-premature infants. *Journal of Pediatrics & Child Health, 35*(5), A2.

Skellern, C.Y., Rogers, Y., & O'Callaghan, M. (2001). A parent-completed developmental questionnaire: Follow up of ex-premature infants. *Journal of Paediatrics & Child Health, 37*(2), 125–129.

Squires, J. (1996). Parent-completed developmental questionnaires: A low-cost strategy for Child Find and screening. *Infants and Young Children, 9*(1), 16–28.

Squires, J., & Bricker, D. (1991). Impact of completing infant developmental questionnaires on at-risk mothers. *Journal of Early Intervention, 15*(2), 162–172.

Squires, J., Bricker, D., & Potter, L. (1997). Revision of a parent-completed developmental screening tool: Ages and Stages Questionnaires. *Journal of Pediatric Psychology, 22*(3), 313–328.

Squires, J., Carter, A., & Kaplan, P. (2003). Developmental monitoring of children conceived by intracytoplasmic sperm injection and in vitro fertilization. *Fertility and Sterility, 79*(2), 453–454.

Squires, J., Katzev, A., & Jenkins, F. (2002, June). Early screening for developmental delays: Use of parent-completed questionnaires in Oregon's Healthy Start Program. *Early Child Development and Care, 172*(3), 275–282.

Squires, J., Nickel, R., & Bricker, D. (1990). Use of parent-completed developmental questionnaires for Child-Find and screening. *Infants and Young Children, 3*(2), 46–57.

Squires, J., Nickel, R., & Eisert, E. (1996). Early detection of developmental problems: Strategies for monitoring young children in the practice setting. *Journal of Developmental and Behavioral Pediatrics, 17*(6), 410–427.

Squires, J., Potter, L., Bricker, D., & Lamorey, S. (1998). Parent-completed developmental questionnaires: Effectiveness with low and middle income parents. *Early Childhood Research Quarterly, 13*(2), 347–356.

Sturner, R., Layton, T., Evans, A., Funk, S., & Machon, M. (1994). Preschool speech and language screening: A review of currently available tests. *Topics in Early Childhood Special Education, 12*(2), 25–36.

Werner, E.E., & Smith, R.S. (1992). *Overcoming the odds: High risk children from birth to adulthood.* Ithaca, NY: Cornell University Press.

Williams, D.L., Gelijns, A.C., Moskowitz, A.J., Weinberg, A.D., Ng, J.H., Crawford, E., et al. (2000, April). Hypoplastic left heart syndrome: Valuing the survival. *Journal of Thoracic and Cardiovascular Surgery, 119*(4, Pt. 1), 720–731.

B

Glossary

ASQ™

This glossary contains definitions of terminology used in this volume to discuss the screening of children.

Corrected age A chronological date correction for weeks of prematurity when the actual date of birth is more than 3 weeks earlier than the expected birthdate. To calculate a corrected age, the weeks of prematurity are subtracted from the infant's chronological age.

Chronological age – number of weeks premature = corrected age

For example, a child who was born 8 weeks prematurely and whose chronological age is 60 weeks will be given a corrected age of 52 weeks. The authors recommend that the corrected age be used until the infant reaches 24 months of age.

Corrected date of birth (CDOB) A chronological date correction for weeks of prematurity when the actual date of birth is more than 3 weeks earlier than the expected birthdate. To calculate CDOB, add the weeks of prematurity to the child's date of birth.

Cutoff point Empirically derived score that indicates when a child's performance is suspect and referral for further assessment is appropriate.

Developmental assessment Establishes baseline, or entry level of measurement, of a child's skills across developmental areas (e.g., communication, gross motor, fine motor, problem solving, personal-social).

Identified Also known as *screened.* Descriptive of children whose score on a screening tool, such as the *Ages & Stages Questionnaires,* falls below the cutoff score, and who are identified as needing further assessment.

Monitoring Periodic developmental screening of young children.

Overreferral (or overidentification) Also known as *overscreening.* The proportion of children incorrectly identified as in need of further assessment by the screening tool.

Percent agreement The proportion of agreement between the screening tool and standardized assessments.

Percent screened The percentage of children who are identified as needing further assessment by a screening tool.

Positive predictive value The probability that a child identified by the screening tool as needing further assessment will have intervention needs.

Psychometric study Research examining the validity, reliability, and utility of an assessment instrument.

Reliability Consistency of test scores over time and between testers; the extent to which it is possible to generalize from one test result conducted by one person to test results conducted at different times or by different observers.

Screening A brief procedure to determine whether a child requires further and more comprehensive evaluation.

Sensitivity The proportion of children correctly identified as needing further assessment by the screening tool and who perform below the expected level on a standardized assessment or assessment battery.

Specificity The proportion of children correctly excluded as developing typically by the screening tool and who perform at the expected level on a standardized assessment.

Tracking Periodic and sequential developmental screening and referral of young children for intervention services.

Underreferral (or underidentification) Also known as *underscreening.* The proportion of children incorrectly identified as developing typically by the screening tool.

Validity Extent to which a test measures what its authors claim it measures; appropriateness of the inferences that can be made on test results.

C

Sample Forms and Letters—Spanish Version

Ejemplos de formularios y cartas—Versión en español

ASQ™

Throughout this volume, a number of sample forms, as well as letters to the parents and physicians of children participating in an ASQ monitoring program, are provided. To assist program staff who serve Spanish-speaking families, these samples have been translated into Spanish and are provided in this appendix. Staff are granted permission to photocopy these samples and to modify them to suit the needs of their program and the families they serve. The *Ages & Stages Questionnaires* are available in Spanish as well. *Edades y Etapas CD-ROM* contains all of the ASQ questionnaires and the intervention activities (see Appendix D) in Spanish.

A lo largo de este volumen, se provee varios ejemplos de formularios además de ejemplos de cartas a los padres y a los médicos de los niños que participan en el programa. Para ayudar a los proveedores del programa que sirven a las familias hispanohablantes, estos formularios y cartas aparecen traducidos en español en este apéndice. Es permitido fotocopiar y modificarlos para mejor acomodar las necesidades individuales del programa y a las familias que sirven. Se puede conseguir el *Cuestionario de edades y etapas* en español también. *Edades y Etapas CD-ROM* incluye todos los cuestionarios y las actividades de intervencíon (véase Appendix D) en español.

Estimados [fill in parents' or guardians' names]:

Los primeros años en la vida de su hijo/a son muy importantes, porque es el período que lo/a preparara para el triunfo escolar y el resto de su vida. Durante su infancia y su niñez, muchas experiencias deben ser adquiridas y muchas nuevas habilidades aprendidas. Es importante asegurarse de que el progreso de desarrollamiento en cada bebé avance sin ningún problema durante esta etapa; por eso, estamos interesados en ayudar en el desarrollamiento de su bebé. Ustedes nos pueden ayudar al completar el siguiente cuestionario que les llegará por correo en intervalos de 2, 4, o 6 meses. Se les harán preguntas acerca de algunas de las cosas que pueda, o no pueda hacer su bebé, y por favor devuelva tal cuestionario a [fill in staff member's name].

Si el cuestionario completado nos indica que su bebé se está desarrollando sin ningún problema, les enviaremos una carta indicándoles que el desarrollo de su bebé aparenta ser típico para su etapa infantil. Entonces les enviaremos el próximo nivel de preguntas apropiadas para la próxima etapa de desarrollo.

Si nosotros tenemos algo que concerna su bebé, nos pondremos en contacto directamente, y quizás en este momento ustedes querrán consultar a otro doctor o agencia para que conduzcan más examinaciones. Toda información adquirida sobre su bebé y su familia será mantenida en la confidencia más estricta.

Sinceramente,

[fill in staff member's name]
[fill in program name]

A sample information and agreement letter to parents or guardians. This letter should be modified by personnel to reflect the ASQ method(s) to be used by the program.

_____ He leído la descripción del programa que servirá de monitor, y deseo participar. Estoy dispuesto/a a llenar el cuestionario acerca del desarrollo de mi bebé y los devolveré con prontitud.

_____ He leído la descripción del proyecto monitorial. Comprendo el propósito de este programa y no deseo participar.

Firmas de los padres: ____________________

Fecha: ____________________

Nombre del bebé: ____________________

Peso de nacimiento: ____________________

Nombre del doctor del bebé: ____________________

A sample participation agreement to be signed by a child's parents or guardians before beginning implementation procedures (see Chapter 5).

Información de la Familia

1. Número de identificación de su hijo/a ____________
2. Nombre de su hijo/a ____________
   Nombre de los padres (apellido, nombre) ____________
3. Su dirección ____________
   ____
   Código/Zona postal ____________
   Teléfono ____________
4. Fecha de nacimiento _____/_____/_____
5. ¿Sexo? (hijo = 1, hija = 2) ____________
6. ¿Cuánto tiempo estaba embarazada (por semanas)? ________
7. Peso del recién nacido ____________
8. Étnicidad de su hijo/a: ____________

---

9. ¿Necesitaba su bebé cuidado intensivo? (1 = sí, 2 = no) ________
   ¿Cuánto tiempo? (en días) ____________
10. Fecha de entrada en el programa (mes, día, año) _____/_____/_____
11. Estado de su hijo/a
    ¿A riesgo? (1 = sí, 2 = no) ____________
    Si Ud. ha respondido afirmativamente, escriba 3 factores para cada categoría:
    Factores de riesgo medicos ____________
    Factores de riesgo del medioambiente (véase los códigos) ____________
    ¿Tiene su bebé problemas físicos? (1 = sí, 2 = no) ___ Incapacidad ____________
12. Es una familia adoptiva? (1 = sí, 2 = no) ____________

---

13. ¿Cuántos años tenía Ud. (madre) cuándo nació su bebé? ________
14. Apellido paternal de la madre: ____________
15. ¿Están casados? ____________
16. Ganador principal de salario ____________
17. ¿Hasta qué año completó la madre la escuela? ____________
18. ¿Hasta qué año completó el padre la escuela? ____________
19. ¿Qué tipo de trabajo hace la madre? ____________
20. ¿Qué tipo de trabajo hace el padre? ____________
21. ¿Cuánto ganan al año? ____________

---

22. El médico del niño ____________
    Teléfono del médico ____________
23. ¿Fecha esperada del parto? ____________
24. ¿Tuvo el niño cualquier problema médico? ____________
    Si es afirmativa explique ____________
25. ¿Ha tenido el niño cualquier problema médico desde entonces? ____________
26. ¿Cuántos niños viven en su hogar? ____________

A sample Child and Family Demographic Information Sheet. This form or one like it should be easily accessible throughout the child's involvement in the program.

El Bebé y su Familia
Información Demográfica

1. Número de identificación ______________
2. Nombre del bebé ______________
   Nombres de los padres/guardianes (apellido, nombre) ______________
3. Domicilio: Número, calle ______________
   Ciudad ______________
   Condado ______________ Estado ______________ Código postal ______________
   Teléfono: Domicilio ______________
   Trabajo ______________
4. Fecha de nacimiento del bebé (mes/día/año) _____/_____/_____
5. Sexo del bebé (varón, hembra) ______________
6. Fecha de admisión en el programa (mes/día/año) _____/_____/_____
7. Estado civil de los padres ______________
8. Persona con el salario principal ______________
9. Nivel educacional más alto de la madre ______________
10. Nivel educacional más alto del padre ______________
11. Ocupación de la madre ______________
12. Ocupación del padre ______________
13. Estimado salario anual de la familia ______________
14. Número total de menores en la familia ______________

A sample Child and Family Demographic Information Update Sheet. A form like this should be completed as necessary throughout the child's involvement in the program.

Número de identificación ______________

Sumario Informativo del Bebé

1. Nombre del bebé ______________
2. Fecha de nacimiento del bebé (mes, día, año) _____/_____/_____
3. Tiempo en embarazo (en semanas) ______________
4. Corrección de fecha de nacimiento prematuro (si aplicable) ______________
5. Nombre de la madre ______________
6. Nombre del padre ______________
7. Otros guardianes ______________
8. Domicilio: Número, calle ______________
   Ciudad ______________
   Condado ______________ Estado ______________ Código postal ______________
   Teléfono: Domicilio ______________
   Trabajo ______________
9. Nombre del doctor ______________
   Número, calle ______________
   Ciudad ______________
   Condado ______________ Estado ______________ Código postal ______________
   Teléfono ______________
10. Notas/comentarios ______________

The Child Information Summary Sheet should be completed during the first step of the implementation phase. It should be kept in the child's file.

Estimados [fill in parents' or guardians' names]:

Muchas gracias por la participación de su hijo/a en *Edades y Etapas: Un Cuestionario Completado por los Padres para Evaluar a los Niños* en la sesión de juego de los doce meses. Encontramos que el desarrollo de su hijo/a se encuentra dentro de los niveles normales para su edad.

Esperamos que Ud. y su hijo/a hayan disfrutado la experiencia. También esperamos con gusto que continúe su apoyo en este proyecto. Recibirá otro cuestionario una semana antes que su hijo/a cumpla 16 meses. Favor llámenos si tiene alguna pregunta.

¡Muchas Gracias!

[fill in staff member's name]
[fill in program name]

A sample feedback letter to parents or guardians whose children's questionnaire scores indicate typical development.

Estimados padres:

Quisieramos que tomasen unos minutos para evaluar nuestro cuestionario. Apreciamos muchísimo su participación en nuestro programa, y esperamos que nuestro servicio les haya ayudado.

Por favor marque el número que exprese mejor su opinión

1. Aproximadamente, ¿cuántos minutos se demoraron en terminar cada cuestionario? _____ minutos. Consideran que este tiempo fue:

muy poco tiempo — mucho tiempo

1 2 3 4

Comentarios:

2. ¿El cuestionario les llamó la atención a habilidades o actividades que su bebé pudo hacer que Uds. hasta ahora no estaban seguros?

pocas — muchas

1 2 3 4

Comentarios:

3. Después de completar los cuestionarios, ¿les crearon nuevas ideas de como reciprocar o jugar con su bebé?

pocas — muchas

1 2 3 4

Comentarios:

4. ¿Hubo alguna pregunta que no estuvo muy clara o estuvo difícil de comprender?

pocas — muchas

1 2 3 4

Comentarios:

5. ¿Ha disfrutado de participar en este programa?

poco — mucho

1 2 3 4

Comentarios:

Si tiene algún otro comentario acerca del cuestionario, escríbalos en el reverso de esta página.

An example of a feedback form sent to parents participating in the program. Such a survey should be distributed at least once a year, if possible.

D

Intervention Activities Sheets

ASQ™

The intervention activities in this appendix include games and other fun events for parents and caregivers and their young children. Each sheet contains activities that correspond to ages in the ASQ intervals: 4- to 8-month-olds, 8- to 12-month-olds, 12- to 16-month-olds, 16- to 20-month-olds, 20- to 24-month-olds, 24- to 30-month-olds, 30- to 36-month-olds, 36- to 48-month-olds, 48- to 60-month-olds, and 60- to 66-month-olds. These sheets can be duplicated and used in monitoring programs in a variety of ways. The intervention activities are also available on the *ASQ CD-ROM* (in English) and *Edades y Etapas CD-ROM* (in Spanish).

The intervention activities suggestions can be mailed or given to parents with the *Ages & Stages Questionnaires,* or they can be attached to a feedback letter along with the ASQ results. Parents can be encouraged to post the sheets on their refrigerator door or bulletin board and to try activities with their young children as time allows. If a child has difficulties in a particular developmental area, a service provider can star or underline certain games that might be particularly useful for parents to present. Similarly, service providers and family members can modify the activities to make them match the family's cultural setting and available materials (see pp. 65–66). ***As with all activities for young children, these intervention activities should be supervised by an adult at all times.***

The intervention activities for 4- to 36-month-olds suggested in this appendix were compiled by Davidson, J., & Cripe, J. (1987). *Intervention activities.* Eugene: University of Oregon Infant Monitoring Project.

ACTIVITIES FOR INFANTS 4–8 MONTHS OLD

Put a windup toy beside or behind your baby. Watch to see if your baby searches for the sound.	Give your baby a spoon to grasp and chew on. It's easy to hold and feels good in the mouth. It's also great for banging, swiping, and dropping.	While sitting on the floor, place your baby in a sitting position inside your legs. Use your legs and chest to provide only as much support as your baby needs. This allows you to play with your baby while encouraging independent sitting.	Gently rub your baby with a soft cloth, a paper towel, or nylon. Talk about how things feel (soft, rough, slippery). Lotion feels good, too.	Let your baby see him- or herself in a mirror. Place an unbreakable mirror on the side of your baby's crib or changing table so he or she can watch. Look in the mirror with your baby, too. Smile and wave at your baby.
Make your own crib gym. Attach kitchen tools (measuring spoons and cups, potato masher or whips, shaker cup with a bell inside) to yarn tied across your baby's crib. Place the crib gym where your baby can kick it. *Take it down when your baby is not playing.* Always supervise.	Play voice games. Talk with a high or low voice. Click your tongue. Whisper. Take turns with your baby. Repeat any sounds made by him or her. Place your baby so you are face to face—your baby will watch as you make sounds.	Fill a small plastic bottle (medicine bottle with child-proof cap) with beans or rice. Let your baby shake it to make noise.	Make another shaker using bells. Encourage your baby to hold one in each hand and shake them both. Watch to see if your baby likes one sound better than another.	Place your baby on his or her tummy with favorite toys or objects around but just slightly out of reach. Encourage him or her to reach out for toys and move toward them.
Fill an empty tissue box with strips of paper. Your baby will love pulling them out. (Do not use colored newsprint or magazines; they are toxic. Never use plastic bags or wrap.)	Safely attach a favorite toy to a side of your baby's crib, swing, or cradle chair for her or him to reach and grasp. Change toys frequently to give her or him new things to see and do.	Place your baby in a chair or carseat, or prop him or her up with pillows. Bounce and play with a flowing scarf or a large bouncing ball. Move it slowly up, then down or to the side, so your baby can follow movement with his or her eyes.	With your baby lying on his or her back, place a toy within sight but out of reach, or move a toy across your baby's visual range. Encourage him or her to roll to get the toy.	Play Peekaboo with hands, cloth, or a diaper. Put the cloth over your face first. Then let your baby hide. Pull the cloth off if your baby can't. Encourage her or him to play. Take turns.
Place your baby in a chair or carseat to watch everyday activities. Tell your baby what you are doing. Let your baby see, hear, and touch common objects. You can give your baby attention while getting things done.	Place your baby on your knee facing you. Bounce her or him to the rhythm of a nursery rhyme. Sing and rock with the rhythm. Help your baby bring his or her hands together to clap to the rhythm.	Your baby will like to throw toys to the floor. Take a little time to play this "go and fetch" game. It helps your baby to learn to release objects. Give baby a box or pan to practice dropping toys into.	Once your baby starts rolling or crawling on his or her tummy, play "come and get me." Let your baby move, then chase after her and hug her when you catch her.	Place your baby facing you. Your baby can watch you change facial expressions (big smile, poking out tongue, widening eyes, raising eyebrows, puffing or blowing). Give your baby a turn. Do what your baby does.

ACTIVITIES FOR INFANTS 8–12 MONTHS OLD

Let your baby feed her- or himself. This gives your baby practice picking up small objects (cereal, cooked peas) and also gives him experience with textures in his hands and mouth. Soon your baby will be able to finger feed an entire meal.	Your baby will be interested in banging objects to make noise. Give your baby blocks to bang, rattles to shake, or wooden spoons to bang on containers. Show your baby how to bang objects together.	A good pastime is putting objects in and out of containers. Give your baby plastic containers with large beads or blocks. Your baby may enjoy putting socks in and out of the sock drawer or small cartons (Jell-O, tuna or soup cans) on and off shelves.	Mirrors are exciting at this age. Let your baby pat and poke at herself in the mirror. Smile and make faces together in the mirror.	Your baby will begin using her or his index fingers to poke. Let your baby poke at a play telephone or busy box. Your baby will want to poke at faces. Name the body parts as your baby touches your face.
Put toys on a sofa or sturdy table so your baby can practice standing while playing with the toys.	Find a big box that your baby can crawl in and out of. Stay close by and talk to your baby about what he or she is doing. "You went *in*! Now you are *out*!"	Read baby books or colorful magazines by pointing and telling your baby what is in the picture. Let your baby pat pictures in the book.	Play hide-and-seek games with objects. Let your baby see you hide an object under a blanket, diaper, or pillow. If your baby doesn't uncover the object, just cover part of it. Help your baby find the object.	Play ball games. Roll a ball to your baby. Help your baby, or have a partner help him roll the ball back to you. Your baby may even throw the ball, so beach balls or Nerf balls are great for this game.
Turn on a radio or stereo. Hold your baby in a standing position and let your baby bounce and dance. If your baby can stand with a little support, hold her hands and dance like partners.	Play imitation games like Peekaboo and So Big. Show pleasure at your baby's imitations of movements and sounds. Babies enjoy playing the same games over and over.	Let your baby play with plastic measuring cups, cups with handles, sieves and strainers, sponges, and balls that float in the bathtub. Bath time is a great learning time.	Play Pat-a-cake with your baby. Clap his or her hands together or take turns. Wait and see if your baby signals you to start the game again. Try the game using blocks or spoons to clap and bang with.	Your baby will play more with different sounds like "la-la" and "da-da." Copy the sounds your baby makes. Add a new one and see if your baby tries it, too. Enjoy baby's early attempts at talking.
Make a simple puzzle for your baby by putting blocks or Ping-Pong balls inside a muffin pan or egg carton.	You can make another simple toy by cutting a round hole in the plastic lid of a coffee can. Give your baby wooden clothes pins or Ping-Pong balls to drop inside.	Say "Hi" and wave when entering a room with your baby. Encourage your baby to imitate. Help your baby wave to greet others. Waving "Hi" and "Bye" are early gestures.	Let your baby make choices. Offer two toys or foods and see which one your baby picks. Encourage your baby to reach or point to the chosen object. Babies have definite likes and dislikes!	New places and people are good experiences for your baby, but these can be frightening. Let your baby watch and listen and move at his or her own speed. Go slowly. Your baby will tell you when he or she is ready for more.

ACTIVITIES FOR INFANTS 12–16 MONTHS OLD

Babies love games at this age (Pat-a-cake, This Little Piggy Went to Market). Try different ways of playing the games and see if your baby will try it with you. Hide behind furniture or doors for Peek-aboo; clap blocks or pan lids for Pat-a-cake.	Make puppets out of a sock or paper bag—one for you and one for your baby. Have your puppet talk to your baby or your baby's puppet. Encourage your baby to "talk" back.	To encourage your baby's first steps, hold your baby in standing position, facing another person. Have your baby step toward the other person to get a favorite toy or treat.	Give your baby containers with lids or different compartments filled with blocks or other small toys. Let your baby open and dump. Play "putting things back." This will help your baby learn how to release objects where he or she wants them.	Loosely wrap a small toy in a paper towel or facial tissue without tape. Your baby can unwrap it and find a surprise. Use tissue paper or wrapping paper, too. It's brightly colored and noisy.
Babies enjoy push and pull toys. Make your own pull toy by threading yogurt cartons, spools, or small boxes on a piece of yarn or soft string (about 2 feet long). Tie a bead or plastic stacking ring on one end for a handle.	Tape a large piece of drawing paper to a table. Show your baby how to scribble with large nontoxic crayons. Take turns making marks on the paper. It's also fun to paint with water.	Arrange furniture so your baby can work his or her way around a room by stepping across gaps between furniture. This encourages balance in walking.	Babies continue to love making noise. Make sound shakers by stringing canning rims together or filling medicine bottles (with child-proof caps) with different-sounding objects like marbles, rice, salt, bolts, and so forth. *Be careful to secure lids tightly.*	This is the time your baby learns that adults can be useful! When your baby "asks" for something by vocalizing or pointing, respond to his or her signal. Name the object your baby wants and encourage him or her to communicate again—taking turns with each other in a "conversation."
Play the naming game. Name body parts, common objects, and people. This lets your baby know that everything has a name and helps him or her begin to learn these names.	Make an obstacle course with boxes or furniture so your baby can climb in, on, over, under, and through. A big box can be a great place to sit and play.	Let your baby help you clean up. Play "feed the wastebasket" or "give it to Mommy or Daddy."	Make a surprise bag for your baby to find in the morning. Fill a paper or cloth bag with a soft toy, something to make a sound, a little plastic jar with a screw-top lid, or a book with cardboard pages.	Play "pretend" with a stuffed animal or doll. Show and tell your baby what the doll is doing (walking, going to bed, eating, dancing across a table). See if your baby will make the doll move and do things as you request. Take turns.
Cut up safe finger foods (do not use foods that pose a danger of your baby's choking) in small pieces and allow your baby to feed him- or herself. It is good practice to pick up small things and feel different textures (bananas, soft crackers, berries).	Let your baby "help" during daily routines. Encourage your baby to "get" the cup and spoon for mealtime, to "find" shoes and coat for dressing, and to "bring" the pants or diaper for changing. Following directions is an important skill for your baby to learn.	Your baby is learning that different toys do different things. Give your baby lots of things to roll, push, pull, hug, shake, poke, turn, stack, spin, and stir.	Most babies enjoy music. Clap and dance to the music. Encourage your baby to practice balance by moving forward, around, and back. Hold his or her hands for support, if needed.	Prepare your baby for a future activity or trip by talking about it beforehand. Your baby will feel a part of what is going on rather than being just an observer. It may also help reduce some fear of being "left behind."

ACTIVITIES FOR TODDLERS 16 –20 MONTHS OLD

Toddlers love to play in water. Put "squeezing" objects in the bathtub, such as sponges or squeeze bottles, along with dump-and-pour toys (cups, bowls).	Toddlers are excited about bubbles. Let your toddler try to blow bubbles or watch you blow bubbles through a straw. Bubbles are fun to pop and chase, too.	Pretend play becomes even more fun at this age. Encourage your toddler to have a doll or stuffed toy do what he or she does—walk, go to bed, dance, eat, and jump. Include the doll in daily activities or games.	Make instant pudding together. Let your toddler "help" by dumping pudding, pouring milk, and stirring. The results are good to eat or can be used for finger painting.	Use boxes or buckets for your toddler to throw bean bags or balls into. Practice overhand release of the ball or bean bag.
Play Hide and Seek. Your toddler can hide with another person or by him- or herself for you to find. Then take your turn to hide and let your toddler find you.	Toddlers love movement. Take him or her to the park to ride on rocking toys, swings, and small slides. You may want to hold your toddler in your lap on the swing and on the slide at first.	Sing action songs together such as "Ring Around the Rosey," "Itsy-Bitsy Spider," and "This Is the Way We Wash Our Hands." Do actions together. Move with the rhythm. Wait for your toddler to anticipate the action.	Put favorite toys in a laundry basket slightly out of reach of your toddler or in a clear container with a tight lid. Wait for your toddler to request the objects, giving him or her a reason to communicate. Respond to his or her requests.	Your toddler may become interested in "art activities." Use large nontoxic crayons and a large pad of paper. Felt-tip markers are more exciting with their bright colors. Let your toddler scribble his or her own picture as you make one.
A favorite pull toy often is a small wagon or an old purse for collecting things. Your toddler can practice putting objects in and out of it. It can also be used to store favorite items.	Make a picturebook by putting common, simple pictures cut from magazines into a photo album. Your toddler will enjoy photos of him- or herself and family members. Pictures of pets are favorites, too.	Toddlers are interested in playing with balls. Use a beach ball to roll, throw, and kick.	Play the "What's that?" game by pointing to clothing, toys, body parts, objects, or pictures and asking your toddler to name them. If your toddler doesn't respond, name it for him or her and encourage imitation of the words.	Fill a plastic tub with cornmeal or oatmeal. Put in kitchen spoons, strainer, measuring cups, funnels, or plastic containers. Toddlers can fill, dump, pour, and learn about textures and use of objects as tools. Tasting won't be harmful.
Toddlers will begin putting objects together. Simple puzzles (separate pieces) with knobs are great. Putting keys into locks and letters into mailbox slots is fun, too.	Get two containers (coffee cups or cereal bowls) that look the same and a small toy. Hide the toy under one container while your toddler watches. Ask him or her, "Where did it go?" Eventually you can play the "old shell game."	Help your toddler sort objects into piles. He or she can help you sort laundry (put socks in one pile and shirts in another). Play "clean up" games. Have your toddler put toys on specified shelves or boxes.	Save milk cartons, Jell-O boxes, or pudding boxes. Your toddler can stack them to make towers. You can also stuff grocery bags with newspapers and tape them shut to make big blocks.	Lay out your toddler's clothes on the bed before dressing. Ask him or her to give you a shirt, pants, shoes, and socks. This is an easy way to learn the names of common items.

ACTIVITIES FOR TODDLERS 20–24 MONTHS OLD

Toddlers enjoy looking at old pictures of themselves. Tell simple stories about her or him as you look at the pictures. Talk about what was happening when the picture was taken.	Cut a rectangular hole in the top of a shoebox. Let your toddler insert an old deck of playing cards or used envelopes. The box is easy storage for your toddler's "mail."	Set up your own bowling game using plastic tumblers, tennis ball cans, or empty plastic bottles for bowling pins. Show your toddler how to roll the ball to knock down the pins. Then let your toddler try.	Many everyday items (socks, spoons, shoes, mittens) can help your toddler learn about matching. Hold up an object, and ask if he or she can find one like yours. Name the objects while playing the game.	Hide a loudly ticking clock or a softly playing transistor radio in a room and have your child find it. Take turns by letting him or her hide and you find.
A good body parts song is "Head, Shoulders, Knees, and Toes." Get more detailed with body parts by naming teeth, eyebrows, fingernails, and so forth.	Make your toddler an outdoor "paint" set by using a large wide paint brush and a bowl or bucket of water. Your toddler will have fun "painting" the side of the house, a fence, or the front porch.	Turn objects upside down (books, cups, shoes) and see if your toddler notices they're wrong and turns them back the right way. Your toddler will begin to enjoy playing "silly" games.	Give your toddler some of your old clothes (hats, shirts, scarves, purses, necklaces, sunglasses) to use for dress up. Make sure your toddler sees him- or herself in the mirror. Ask him or her to tell you who is all dressed up.	Use plastic farm animals or stuffed animals to tell the Old McDonald story. Use sound effects!
Make grocery sack blocks by filling large grocery sacks about half full with shredded or crumpled newspaper. Fold the top of the sack over and tape it shut. Your toddler will enjoy tearing and crumpling the paper and stuffing the sacks. The blocks are great for stacking and building. *Avoid newsprint contact with mouth. Wash hands after this activity.*	"Dress up" clothes offer extra practice for putting on and taking off shirts, pants, shoes, and socks. Toddlers can fasten big zippers and buttons.	Put small containers, spoons, measuring cups, funnels, a bucket, shovels, and a colander into a sandbox. Don't forget to include cars and trucks to drive on sand roads.	Rhymes and songs with actions are popular at this age. "Itsy-Bitsy Spider," "I'm a Little Teapot," and "Where Is Thumbkin?" are usual favorites. Make up your own using your toddler's name in the song.	Make your own playdough by mixing 2 cups flour and $^3/_4$ cup salt. Add $^1/_2$ cup water and 2 tablespoons salad oil. Knead well until it's smooth; add food coloring, and knead until color is fully blended. Toddlers will love squishing, squeezing, and pounding the dough.
Playing beside or around other children the same age is fun but usually requires adult supervision. Trips to the park are good ways to begin practicing interacting with other children.	Play the "show me" game when looking at books. Ask your toddler to find an object in a picture. Take turns. Let your toddler ask you to find an object in a picture. Let him or her turn the pages.	Add a few Ping-Pong balls to your toddler's bath toys. Play a "pop up" game by showing your toddler how balls pop back up after holding them under the water.	Clean plastic containers with push or screw-on lids are great places to "hide" a favorite object or treat. Toddlers will practice pulling and twisting them to solve the "problem" of getting the object. Watch to see if your toddler asks you to help.	Make a book by pasting different textures on each page. Materials such as sandpaper, feathers, cotton balls, nylon, silk, and buttons lend themselves to words such as *rough, smooth, hard,* and *soft.*

ACTIVITIES FOR CHILDREN 24–30 MONTHS OLD

Add actions to your child's favorite nursery rhymes. Easy action rhymes include "Here We Go 'Round the Mulberry Bush," "Jack Be Nimble," "This Is the Way We Wash Our Clothes," "Ring Around the Rosey," and "London Bridge."	Play Target Toss with a large bucket or box and bean bags or balls. Help your child count how many he or she gets in the target. A ball of yarn or rolled-up socks also work well for an indoor target game.	Wrap tape around one end of a piece of yarn to make it stiff like a needle and put a large knot at the other end. Have your child string large elbow macaroni, buttons, spoons, or beads. Make an edible necklace out of Cheerios.	Children at this age love outings. One special outing can be going to the library. The librarian can help you find appropriate books. Make a special time for reading (like bedtime stories).	Play a jumping game when you take a walk by jumping over the cracks in the sidewalk. You may have to hold your child and help him or her jump over at first.
Take time to draw with your child when he or she wants to get out paper and crayons. Draw large shapes and let your child color them in. Take turns.	During sandbox play, try wetting some of the sand. Show your child how to pack the container with the wet sand and turn it over to make sand structures or cakes.	Add an old catalog or two to your child's library. It's a good "picture" book for naming common objects.	Give your child soap, a washcloth, and a dishpan of water. Let your child wash a "dirty" doll, toy dishes, or doll clothes. It's good practice for hand washing and drying.	Make "sound" containers using plastic Easter eggs or L'eggs eggs. Fill eggs with noisy objects like sand, beans, or rice and tape the eggs shut. Have two eggs for each sound. Help your child match sounds and put them back in the carton together.
Show your child how to make snakes, balls, or roll-out pancakes with a small rolling pin using Play-Doh. Use large cookie cutters to make new Play-Doh shapes.	Children at this age love to pretend and really enjoy it when you can pretend with them. Pretend you are different animals, like a dog or cat. Make animal sounds and actions. Let your child be the pet owner who pets and feeds you.	Your child will begin to be able to make choices. Help her or him choose what to wear each day by giving a choice between two pairs of socks, two shirts, and so forth. Give choices at other times like snack or mealtime (two kinds of drink, cracker, etc.).	Enhance listening skills by playing cassettes with both slow and fast music. Songs with speed changes are great. Show your child how to move fast or slow with the music. (You might find children's cassettes at your local library.)	Children can find endless uses for boxes. A box big enough for your child to fit in can become a car. An appliance box with holes cut for windows and a door can become your child's playhouse. Decorating the boxes with crayons, markers, or paints can be a fun activity to do together.
Play "Follow the Leader." Walk on tiptoes, walk backward, and walk slow or fast with big steps and little steps.	Try a new twist to fingerpainting. Use whipping cream on a washable surface (cookie sheet, Formica table). Help your child spread it around and draw pictures with your fingers. Add food coloring to give it some color.	Action is an important part of a child's life. Play a game with a ball where you give directions and your child does the actions, such as "*roll* the ball." *Kick, throw, push, bounce,* and *catch* are other good actions. Take turns giving the directions.	Make an obstacle course using chairs, pillows, or large cartons. Tell your child to crawl over, under, through, behind, in front of, or between the objects. Be careful arranging so the pieces won't tip and hurt your child.	Collect little and big things (balls, blocks, plates). Show and describe (big/little) the objects. Ask your child to give you a big ball, then all the big balls. Do the same for *little.* Another big/little game is making yourself big by stretching your arms up high and making yourself little by squatting down.

ACTIVITIES FOR CHILDREN 30 – 36 MONTHS OLD

Tell or read a familiar story and pause frequently to leave out a word, asking your child to "fill it in." For example, Little Red Riding Hood said, "Grandmother, what big ________ you have."	Teach somersaults by doing one yourself first. Then help your child do one. Let him or her try it alone. Make sure furniture is out of the way. You may want to put some pillows on the floor for safety.	Give a cup to your child. Use bits of cereal or fruit and place one in your child's cup ("one for you") and one in your cup ("one for me"). Take turns. Dump out your child's cup and help count the pieces. This is good practice for early math skills.	Put an old blanket over a table to make a tent or house. Pack a "picnic" sack for your camper. Have your child take along a pillow on the "camp out" for a nap. Flashlights are especially fun.	Get a piece of butcher paper large enough for your child to lie on. Draw around your child's body to make an outline. Don't forget fingers and toes. Talk about body parts and print the words on the paper. Let your child color the poster. Hang the poster on a wall in your child's room.
Children at this age may be interested in creating art in different ways. Try cutting a potato in half and carving a simple shape or design for your child to dip in paint and then stamp onto paper.	Add water to tempera paint to make it runny. Drop some paint on a paper and blow through a straw to move the paint around the paper, or fill an old roll-on deodorant bottle with watered-down paint. Your child can roll color onto the paper.	A good activity to learn location words is to build roads and bridges with blocks. Use toy cars to go on the road, under or over a bridge, between the houses, and so forth.	Trace around simple objects with your child. Use cups of different sizes, blocks, or your child's and your hands. Using felt-tip markers or crayons of different colors makes it even more fun.	Have your child help you set the table. First, have your child place the plates, then glasses, and then napkins. By placing one at each place, he or she will learn one-to-one correspondence. Show your child where the utensils should be placed.
Collect empty boxes (cereal, TV dinners, egg cartons) and help your child set up his or her own grocery store.	Help your child learn new words to describe objects in everyday conversations. Describe by color, size, and shape (the *blue* cup, the *big* ball). Also, describe how things move (a car goes *fast*, a turtle moves *slowly*) and how they feel (ice cream is *cold*, soup is *hot*).	Make your own puzzles by cutting out magazine pictures of whole people. Have your child help glue pictures onto cardboard. Cut pictures into three pieces by cutting curvy lines. Head, trunk, and legs make good pieces for your child to put together.	Dribble different colors of paint in the middle or on one side of a paper. Fold the paper in half. Let your child open the paper to see the design it makes.	A good game for trips in the car is to play a matching game with a set of Old Maid cards. Place a few different cards in front of your child. Give him or her a card that matches one displayed and ask him or her to find the card like the one you gave him or her.
Cut pictures out of magazines to make two groups such as dogs, food, toys, or clothes. Have two boxes ready and put a picture of a dog in one and of food in the other. Have your child put additional pictures in the right box, helping him or her learn about categories.	Cut a stiff paper plate to make a hand paddle and show your child how to use it to hit a balloon. See how long your child can keep the balloon in the air or how many times he or she can hit it back to you. This activity helps develop large body and eye–hand coordination. Always carefully supervise when playing with balloons.	To improve coordination and balance, show your child the "bear walk" by walking on hands and feet, keeping the legs and arms straight. Try the "rabbit hop" by crouching down and then jumping forward.	Encourage your child to try the "elephant walk," bending forward at the waist and letting your arms (hands clasped together) swing freely while taking slow and heavy steps. This is great to do with music.	Make a poster of your child's favorite things using pictures from old magazines. Use safety scissors and paste or a glue stick to allow your child to do it independently, yet safely.

ACTIVITIES FOR CHILDREN 36 – 48 MONTHS OLD

Make a book "about me" for your child. Save family pictures, leaves, magazine pictures of a favorite food, and drawings your child makes. Put them in a photo album, or glue onto sheets of paper and staple together to make a book.	Make a bird feeder using peanut butter and bird seed. Help your child find a pine cone or a piece of wood to spread peanut butter on. Roll in or sprinkle with seeds and hang in a tree or outside a window. While your child watches the birds, ask her about the number, size, and color of the different birds that visit.	Grow a plant. Choose seeds that sprout quickly (beans or peas), and together with your child place the seeds in a paper cup, filling almost to the top with dirt. Place the seeds $\frac{1}{2}$ inch under the soil. Put the cup in a sunny windowsill and encourage your child to water and watch the plant grow.	Before bedtime, look at a magazine or children's book together. Ask your child to point to pictures as you name them, such as "Where is the truck?" Be silly and ask him to point with his elbow or foot. Ask him to show you something that is round or something that goes fast.	Play a matching game. Find two sets of 10 or more pictures. You can use pictures from two copies of the same magazine or a deck of playing cards. Lay the pictures face up and ask your child to find two that are the same. Start with two picture sets and gradually add more.
While cooking or eating dinner, play the "more or less" game with your child. Ask who has *more* "potatoes" and who has *less*. Try this using same-size glasses or cups, filled with juice or milk.	Cut out some large paper circles and show them to your child. Talk with your child about things in her world that are "round" (a ball, the moon). Cut the circle in half, and ask her if she can make it round again. Next, cut the circle into three pieces, and so forth.	During bath time, play Simon Says to teach your child names of body parts. First, you can be "Simon" and help your child wash the part of his body that "Simon says." Let your child have a turn to be "Simon," too. Be sure to name each body part as it is washed and give your child a chance to wash himself.	Talk about the number *3*. Read stories that have *3* in them (*The Three Billy Goats Gruff, Three Little Pigs, The Three Bears*). Encourage your child to count to 3 using similar objects (rocks, cards, blocks). Talk about being 3 years old. After your child gets the idea, move up to the numbers 4, 5, and so forth as long as your child is interested.	Put out several objects that are familiar to your child (brush, coat, banana, spoon, book). Ask your child to show you which one you can eat or which one you wear outside. Help your child put the objects in groups that go together, such as "things that we eat" and "things that we wear."
When your child is getting dressed, encourage her to practice with buttons and zippers. Play a game of Peekaboo to show her how buttons go through the holes. Pretend the zipper is a choo-choo train going "up and down" the track.	Practice following directions. Play a silly game where you ask your child to do two or three fun or unusual things in a row. For example, ask him to "Touch your elbow and then run in a circle" or "Find a book and put it on your head."	Encourage your child's "sharing skills" by making a play corner in your home. Include only two children to start (a brother, sister, or friend) and have a few of the same type of toys available so the children don't have to share all the time. Puppets or blocks are good because they encourage playing together. If needed, use an egg or oven timer with a bell to allow the children equal time with the toys.	Listen for sounds. Find a cozy spot, and sit with your child. Listen and identify all the sounds that you hear. Ask your child if it is a *loud* or *soft* sound. Try this activity inside and outside your home.	Make an adventure path outside. Use a garden hose, rope, or piece of chalk and make a "path" that goes *under* the bench, *around* the tree, and *along* the wall. Walk your child through the path first, using these words. After she can do it, make a new path or have your child make a path.
Find large pieces of paper or cardboard for your child to draw on. Using crayons, pencils, or markers, play a drawing game where you follow his lead by copying exactly what he draws. Next, encourage him to copy your drawings, such as circles or straight lines.	When reading or telling a familiar story for bedtime, stop and leave out a word. Wait for your child to "fill in the blank."	Make a necklace you can eat by stringing Cheerios or Froot Loops on a piece of yarn or string. Wrap a short piece of tape around the end of the string to make a firm tip for stringing.	Listen and dance to music with your child. You can stop the music for a moment and play the "freeze" game where everyone "freezes," or stands perfectly still, until you start the music again. Try to "freeze" in unusual positions for fun.	Make long scarves out of fabric scraps, old dresses, or old shirts by tearing or cutting long pieces. Use material that is lightweight. Hold on to the edge of the scarf, twirl around, run, and jump.

ACTIVITIES FOR CHILDREN 48 – 60 MONTHS OLD

Play the "who, what, and where" game. Ask your child *who* works in a school, *what* is in a school, and *where* is the school. Expand on your child's answers by asking more questions. Ask about other topics, like the library, bus stop, or post office.	When you are setting the table for a meal, play the "what doesn't belong" game. Add a small toy or other object next to the plate and eating utensils. Ask your child if she can tell you what doesn't belong here. You can try this game any time of the day. For example, while brushing your child's hair, set out a brush, barrette, comb, and a "ball."	Let your child help prepare a picnic. Show him what he can use for the picnic (bread, peanut butter, and apples). Lay out sandwich bags and a lunch box, basket, or large plastic bag. Then go have fun on the picnic.	On a rainy day, pretend to open a shoe store. Use old shoes, paper, pencils, and a chair to sit down and try on shoes. You can be the customer. Encourage your child to "write" your order down. Then she can take a turn being the customer and practice trying on and buying shoes.	Play the "guess what will happen" game to encourage your child's problem-solving and thinking skills. For example, during bath time, ask your child, "What do you think will happen if I turn on the hot and cold water at the same time?" or "What would happen if I stacked the blocks to the top of the ceiling?"
Play "bucket hoops." Have your child stand about 6 feet away and throw a medium-size ball at a large bucket or trash can. For fun on a summer day, fill the bucket with water.	Write your child's name often. When he finishes drawing a picture, be sure to put his name on it and say the letters as you write them. If he is interested, encourage him to name and/or to copy the letters. Point out the letters in your child's name throughout the day on cereal boxes, sign boards, and books.	Invite your child to play a counting game. Using a large piece of paper, make a simple game board with a straight path. Use dice to determine the count. Count with your child, and encourage her to hop the game piece to each square, counting as she touches down.	Make a person with Play-Doh or clay using sticks, buttons, toothpicks, beads, and any other small items. Start with a Play-Doh (or clay) head and body and use the objects for arms, legs, and eyes. Ask your child questions about his person.	Encourage your child to learn her full name, address, and telephone number. Make it into a singing or rhyming game for fun. Ask your child to repeat it back to you when you are riding in the car or on the bus.
Cut out three small, three medium, and three large circles. Color each set of circles a different color (or use colored paper for each). Your child can sort the circles by color or by size. You can also ask your child about the different sizes. For example, ask your child, "Which one is smallest?" Try this game using the buttons removed from an old shirt.	Go on a walk and pick up things you find. Bring the items home and help your child sort them into groups. For example, groups can include rocks, paper, or leaves. Encourage your child to start a "collection" of special things. Find a box or special place where he can display his collection.	Play a picture guessing game. Cover a picture in a familiar book with a sheet of paper and uncover a little at a time until your child has guessed the picture.	Let your child help you prepare a meal. She can spread peanut butter and jelly, peel a banana, cut with a butter knife, pour cereal, and add milk (using a small container). Never give her a task involving the stove or oven without careful supervision.	"Write" and mail a letter to a friend or relative. Provide your child with paper, crayons or pencil, and an envelope. Let him draw, scribble, or write; or he can tell you what to write down. When he is finished, let him fold the letter to fit in the envelope, lick, and seal. You can write the address on the front. Be sure to let him decorate the envelope as well. After he has put the stamp on, help him mail the letter.
Play "circus." Find old, colorful clothes and help your child put on a circus show. Provide a rope on the ground for the high wire act, a box to stand on to announce the acts, fun objects for a magic act, and stuffed animals for the show. Encourage your child's imagination and creativity in planning the show. Don't forget to clap.	Take a pack of playing cards and choose four or five matching sets. Lay the cards out face up, and help your child to find the pairs. Talk about what makes the pairs of cards the "same" and "different."	Make bubbles. The recipe is $^{3}/_{4}$ cup dish washing liquid (Dawn or Joy works best) and 8 cups of water. Use straws to blow bubbles on a cookie sheet. Or make a wand by stringing two pieces of a drinking straw onto a string or piece of yarn. Tie the ends of the string together to make a circle. Holding onto the straw pieces, dip the string in the bubble mixture. Pull it out and gently move forward or backward. You should see lovely, big bubbles.	Make a bean bag to catch and throw. Fill the toe of an old sock or pantyhose with $^{3}/_{4}$ cup dry beans. Sew the remaining side or tie off with a rubber band. Play "hot potato" or simply play catch. Encourage your child to throw the ball overhand and underhand.	Pretend to be an animal. Encourage your child to use her imagination and become a kitty. You can ask, "What do kitties like to eat?" or "Where do kitties live?" Play along, and see how far the game can go.

ACTIVITIES FOR CHILDREN 60–66 MONTHS OLD

Make a nature collage. Collect leaves, pebbles, and small sticks from outside and glue them on a piece of cardboard or stiff paper. (Cereal and cracker boxes can be cut up and used as cardboard.)	Practice writing first names of friends, toys, and relatives. Your child may need to trace the letters of these names at first. Be sure to write in large print letters.	Encourage dramatic play. Help your child act out his or her favorite nursery rhyme, cartoon, or story. Use large, old clothes for costumes.	Play simple ball games such as kickball. Use a large (8″–12″) ball, and slowly roll it toward your child. See if your child can kick the ball and run to "first base."	When reading stories to your child, let her make up the ending; or retell favorite stories with "silly" new endings that she makes up.
Let your child help you with simple cooking tasks such as mashing potatoes, making cheese sandwiches, and fixing a bowl of cereal. Afterward, see if she can tell you the order that you followed to cook and mash the potatoes or to get the bread out of the cupboard and put the cheese on it.	Play "20 Questions." Think of an animal. Let your child ask 20 yes/no questions about the animal until he guesses what animal it is. (You may need to help him ask yes/no questions at first.) Now let your child choose an animal and you ask the 20 questions. You can also use other categories such as food, toys, and people.	You can play "license plate count-up" in the car or on the bus. Look for a license plate that begins with a *1*. Then try to find other plates that begin with *2,3,4,* and so forth, up to *10*. When your child can play "count-up," play "count-down," starting with a license plate beginning with *9*, then *8, 7, 6,* and so forth, down to *1*.	Practice pretend play or pantomime. Here are some things to act out: 1) eating hot pizza with stringy cheese; 2) winning a race; 3) finding a giant spider; 4) walking in thick, sticky mud; and 5) making footprints in wet sand.	Make a simple concentration game with two or three pairs of duplicate playing cards (two king of hearts), or make your own cards out of duplicate pictures or magazine ads. Start with two or three pairs of cards. Turn them face down and mix them up. Let your child turn two cards over and see if they match. If they don't, turn the cards face down again. You can gradually increase to playing with more pairs of cards.
Make an obstacle course either inside or outside your home. You can use cardboard boxes for jumping over or climbing through, broomsticks for laying between chairs for "limbo" (going under), and pillows for walking around. Let your child help lay out the course. After a couple of practice tries, have her complete the obstacle course as quickly as possible. Then try hopping or jumping the course.	After washing hands, practice writing letters and numbers in pudding or thinned, mashed potatoes spread on a cookie sheet or cutting board. Licking fingers is allowed!	Play mystery sock. Put a common household item in a sock. Tie off the top of the sock. Have your child feel the sock and guess what is inside. Take turns guessing what's inside.	Make color rhymes. Take turns rhyming a color and a word: blue, shoe; red, bed; yellow, fellow. You can also rhyme with names (Dad, sad; Jack, sack). Take turns with the rhyming.	Make an "I can read" poster. Cut out names your child can read—fast-food restaurant names, names from cereal cartons, and other foods. You can write your child's name, names of relatives and names of friends on pieces of paper and put them on the poster. Add to the poster as your child learns to read more names.
Play "what doesn't belong?" Let your child find the word that doesn't belong in a list of six or seven spoken words. The one that doesn't belong can be the word that doesn't rhyme or the word that is from a different category. Some examples are 1) fly, try, by, *coat*, sigh, my; 2) Sam, *is*, ram, am, spam, ham; 3) red, orange, purple, green, yellow, *beetle*; 4) spoon, fork, *shirt*, pan, spatula, knife. Have your child give three to four words with one that doesn't belong.	Play the "memory" game. Put five or six familiar objects on a table. Have your child close her eyes. Remove one object, and rearrange the rest. Ask your child which object is missing. Take turns finding the missing object.	Make puppets out of ice cream sticks, paper bags, socks, or egg carton cups. Decorate the puppets with yarn, pens, buttons, and colored paper. Make a puppet stage by turning a coffee table or card table on its side and crouching behind the table top. Be the audience while your child puts on a puppet show.	Play the old shell game. Get four cups or glasses that you cannot see through. Find a small ball, object, or edible item such as a raisin or cracker that fits under the cups. Have your child watch as you place the object under one of the cups and move all the cups around. Have your child try to remember which cup the object is under. Have your child take a turn moving the objects while you guess.	Play "mystery sound." Select household items that make distinct sounds such as a clock, cereal box, metal lid (placed on a pan), and potato chip bag. Put a blindfold on your child and have her try to guess which object she heard. Take turns with your child.

E

Materials List

ASQ™

The Materials List specifies toys and other materials needed to complete the ASQ. Each questionnaire interval is listed across the top; necessary materials are listed in the far left column. Under each questionnaire interval, a dot indicates a particular item is needed to complete the questionnaire. Most items listed are portable and can be brought to the home or waiting room. There are a few items (e.g., steps; chair; stroller, shopping cart, or wagon) that are more difficult to transport. For these particular items, other objects may be substituted.

Many programs using the ASQ in a home visit format have assembled toy kits with the assistance of this Materials List. Some of the items listed are likely to be found in a family home (i.e., cup, clothing), but the home visitor may find it useful to bring novel items from a toy kit to encourage child and parent participation. It also may be helpful to parents to have items on this list available in waiting rooms where parents are completing the ASQ.

AGES & STAGES QUESTIONNAIRES MATERIALS LIST

ASQ INTERVAL:	4	6	8	10	12	14	16	18	20	22	24	27	30	33	36	42	48	54	60
Puzzle—six piece interlocking															•	•	•		
Clothing with button/zipper														•	•	•	•	•	•
Clothing—socks, hats, shoes					•		•												
Clothing—coat, jacket, or shirt					•							•	•	•	•	•	•	•	
Clothing—loose fitting pants													•	•					
Baby bottle	•			•	•	•	•	•		•	•								
Book with pictures				•	•	•	•	•	•	•	•		•	•	•	•			
Chair							•	•	•	•		•	•	•	•				
Cheerios or other small food		•	•	•	•	•	•				•								
Scissors—child-safe															•	•	•	•	•
Coloring book																	•	•	
Container (box or bowl)					•	•	•	•											
Cookies or crackers			•	•															
Crib rail or supportive furniture			•	•	•														
Cup			•	•				•	•	•	•								
Doll or stuffed animal					•	•	•	•	•	•	•	•							
Fork									•	•	•	•					•		
Ladder with rungs																•	•		
Ball—large								•	•	•	•	•	•	•	•	•	•	•	•
Ball—small					•	•	•	•		•				•	•	•	•	•	•
Mirror	•	•	•		•		•	•				•	•	•	•	•			
Paper				•	•	•	•	•	•	•	•	•	•	•	•	•	•	•	•
Pencil, marker, or crayon					•	•	•	•	•	•	•	•	•	•	•	•	•	•	•
String or shoelace				•	•					•	•	•	•	•	•				
Bead—1″–2″										•	•	•	•	•	•				
Blocks—1″–2″		•	•			•	•	•	•	•	•	•	•	•	•				
Stroller, shopping cart, or wagon										•	•	•	•	•	•				
Spoon						•	•	•	•	•	•		•	•	•	•	•	•	•
Toy—small, easy to grasp	•	•	•	•	•	•													
Windup toy or jar with lid									•	•	•	•	•	•					
Steps								•	•	•	•	•	•	•	•	•			
Light switch										•	•	•							
Toothbrush and toothpaste																	•	•	
Soap, water, and towel																•		•	•

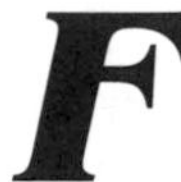

Technical Report on ASQ

This appendix contains information relating to the development and psychometric studies completed on the *Ages & Stages Questionnaires*[1] at the Center on Human Development, University of Oregon, Eugene. First, the development of the ASQ system, including item selection, readability, item analyses, and psychometric studies, is addressed. Second, information about the demographic characteristics of the samples used to study the ASQ system is given. Third, reliability analyses, including internal consistency, alphas, correlation coefficients, and standard error of measurement, are provided. Validity studies are provided fourth, including a description of the determination of the cutoff points, relative operating characteristic (ROC) analysis, concurrent validity, sensitivity, specificity, and overreferral and underreferral rates. The final section of this appendix contains information about risk and nonrisk samples, including performance and effects of risk status.

DEVELOPMENT OF THE *AGES & STAGES QUESTIONNAIRES*

Item Selection

ASQ items were developed using a variety of sources, including standardized developmental tests, nonstandardized tests focused on early development, textbooks, and other literature containing information about early developmental milestones. Using these sources, the following criteria were used to develop items:

1. Skills were selected that could be easily observed or elicited by parents.
2. Skills were selected that were highly likely to occur in a home setting.

Once skills were selected, items were written in familiar, nonjargon wording not to exceed a sixth-grade reading level, illustrations were provided when possible, and concrete examples were provided as appropriate.

Appreciation is extended to Craig Leve for data analysis and to Roland Good for data consultation.

[1]The 60 month questionnaire was in the final stages of development when these studies were conducted. Results of validity studies to date are included.

The five items that make up each developmental area (i.e., communication, gross motor, fine motor, problem solving, and personal-social) were chosen to represent as closely as possible the developmental quotient (DQ) range of 75–100. This range was chosen for two reasons. First, many standardized tests use 1.5–2.0 standard deviations below the mean as the lower end of the typical developmental range; therefore, it was reasoned that any child who was generally unable to perform items at a developmental quotient of 75 should be referred for further assessment. For example, Knobloch, Stevens, and Malone (1980), in assigning diagnostic categories for the Revised Gesell and Amatruda Developmental and Neurological Examination, designated a developmental quotient of 75 or less as the cutoff for atypical test scores. Second, it was reasoned that items above a developmental quotient of 100 would primarily identify children whose development was clearly within typical limits and, thus, the inclusion of such items would add little in attempting to identify children whose development was suspect. Limiting the questionnaires to the developmental range of 75–100 also assisted in maintaining the brevity of the questionnaires.[2]

In order to determine the developmental quotient for each item, the following formula was used:

$$\frac{\text{age equivalence}}{\text{test interval of item}} \times 100 = \text{DQ}$$

The age equivalence was obtained from the source(s) of the item such as the Gesell (Knobloch et al., 1980), the Bayley Scales of Infant Development (Bayley, 1969), and *Developmental Resources: Behavioral Sequences for Assessment and Program Planning* (Cohen & Gross, 1979). When sources varied, a developmental range was used. Table 1 contains the developmental quotient and age equivalent for each item by area for each of the 19 questionnaires. An examination of Table 1 indicates that each area has two items with developmental quotients of approximately 75 (range: 69–77), two items with developmental quotients of approximately 85 (range: 80–92), and two items with developmental quotients of approximately 100 (range: 91–120).

Reading Level

The *Ages & Stages Questionnaires* were designed to be used with a range of parents (e.g., varying income and educational levels); therefore, the reading level ranges between the fourth- and sixth-grade levels, and illustrations were added when possible to clarify items. To ascertain the reading level of the questionnaires, the MinNesota Interactive Readability Approximation Program (MECCA, n.d.) was used, which performed several common readability tests including the Dale-Chall, Raygor, and Fry indexes. Readability levels of the questionnaires ranged from fourth to sixth grade on these three measures, depending on the questionnaire interval and index, with a mean 5.8 grade level across age intervals and indexes.

[2]One "validity check" item with an approximate developmental quotient of 125–150 was also included in each area on the initial version of the ASQ.

Table 1. Age equivalent and developmental quotient of items by area for each questionnaire

Questionnaire items	Communication		Gross motor		Fine motor		Problem solving		Personal-social	
	Age	DQ	Age	DQ	Age	DQ	Age	DQ	Age	DQ
4 Month										
1	12w[a,b]	75	12w	75	12w	75	8–12w	75	12w	75
2	12–16w[c]	75–100	12w	75	12w	75	12w	75	12w	75
3	12–16w	75–100	8–12w	75	12w	75	12w	75	12w	75
4	16w	100	16w	100	16w	100	16w	100	16w	100
5	16w	100	16w	100	16w	100	16w	100	16w	100
6	16w	100	16w	100	16w	100	16w	100	16w	100
6 Month										
1	16w	62	20w	77	20w	77	20w	77	20w	77
2	20w	77	20w	77	20w	77	20w	77	20w	77
3	24w	92	24w	92	24w	92	24w	92	24w	92
4	24w	92	24w	92	24w	92	24w	92	24w	92
5	28w	107	28w	107	28w	107	28w	107	28w	107
6	28w	107	28w	107	28w	107	28w	107	28w	107
8 Month										
1	24w	69	24w	69	24w	69	24w	69	24w	69
2	24w	69	24w	69	24w	69	24w	69	24w	69
3	28w	80	28w	80	28w	80	28w	80	28w	80
4	28w	80	28w	80	28w	80	28w	80	28w	80
5	32w	91	28–32w	80–91	32w	91	32w	91	32w	91
6	32w	91	32w	91	36w	103	32w	91	32w	91
10 Month										
1	28w	70	28w	70	28w	70	28w	70	28w	70
2	28w	70	28–32w	70–80	32w	80	32w	80	32w	80
3	32w	80	32w	80	36w	90	32w	80	32w	80
4	40w	100	40w	100	40w	100	40w	100	40w	100
5	44w	110	40w	100	40w	100	40w	100	40w	100
6	44w	110	44w	110	44w	110	44w	110	44w	110

(continued)

[a]Numbers were rounded to the nearest whole numbers.

[b]w = weeks.

[c]Ranges are presented when the age and developmental quotient (DQ) of an item differed according to developmental sources.

[d]m = months.

Table 1. *(continued)*

Questionnaire items	Communication		Gross motor		Fine motor		Problem solving		Personal-social	
	Age	DQ	Age	DQ	Age	DQ	Age	DQ	Age	DQ
12 Month										
1	40w	77	40w	77	40w	77	40w	77	40w	77
2	44w	85	40w	77	40w	77	40w	77	40w	77
3	44w	85	44w	85	44w	85	44w	85	44w	85
4	48w	92	44w	85	48w	92	44w	85	44w	85
5	52w	100	48w	92	48w	92	48w	92	48w	92
6	52w	100	52w	100	52w	100	52w	100	52w	100
14 Month										
1	44w	80	44w	79	48w	86	44w	79	44w	79
2	52w	93	48w	86	48w	86	48w	86	48w	86
3	52w	93	52w	93	52w	93	52w	93	52w	93
4	52w	93	52–56w	93–100	56w	100	52w	93	56–60w	100–107
5	52w	93	52w	93	60w	107	52w	93	48–60w	86–107
6	56w	100	56w	100	60w	107	56w	100	52–56w	93–100
16 Month										
1	52w	75	52w	75	52w	75	52w	75	15m[d]	93.75
2	52w	75	56w	81.25	52w	75	52w	75	12–15m	75–94
3	52w	75	52w	75	56w	81.25	56w	81	52w	75
4	56w	81.25	56w	81.25	15m	93.75	56w	81	52w	75
5	15m	93.75	15m	93.75	15m	93.75	15m	93.75	12m	94
6	56w	81.25	15m	93.75	18m	112.5	15m	93.75	15m	94
18 Month										
1	56w	74	52w	68	52w	68	56w	74	52w	68
2	56w	74	56w	74	56w	74	56w	74	52w	68
3	56w	74	65w	85	65w	85	65w	85	65w	85
4	65w	85	15m	83	15m	83	65w	85	15m	83
5	78w	108	18m	100	78w	102	78w	102	78w	102
6	91w	126	18m	100	18m	100	78w	102	78w	102

20 Month										
1	15m	75	75w	75	15m	75	15m	75	15m	75
2	15m	75	15m	75	15m	75	18m	90	15m	75
3	18m	90	18m	90	18m	90	20m	100	18m	90
4	18m	90	18m	90	18m	90	20m	100	18m	90
5	21m	105	21m	105	21m	105	<21m	<105	21m	105
6	21m	105	21m	105	18–24m	90–120	24m	120	21m	105
22 Month										
1	13m	70	18m	82	18m	82	13m	70	18m	82
2	21m	95	18–21m	82–95	21m	95	18m	82	21m	95
3	21m	95	15m	85	18–24m	82–109	20m	91	21m	95
4	18–21m	82–95	65w	83	18m	82	20m	91	18–21m	82–95
5	18–21m	85	24m	109	21–29m	95–132	<21m	<91	21m	95
6	24m	109	24m	109	24m	109	24m	109	24m	109
24 Month										
1	18m	75	18m	75	18m	75	18m	75	18m	75
2	18m	75	18m	75	18m	75	18m	75	18m	75
3	21m	87.5	21m	87.5	18–24m	75–100	20m	83	21m	87.5
4	21m	87.5	21m	87.5	21–29m	87.5–121	20m	83	21m	87.5
5	24m	100	24m	100	24m	100	24m	100	24m	100
6	24m	100	24m	100	24m	100	24m	100	24m	100
27 Month										
1	21m	78	21m	78	21m	78	20m	74	21m	78
2	21m	78	21m	78	21–29m	78–107	20m	74	21m	78
3	24m	89	24m	89	24m	89	21m	78	21m	78
4	24m	89	24m	89	24m	89	24m	89	24m	89
5	24m	89	24m	89	24m	89	24m	89	24m	89
6	30m	111	30m	111	30m	111	30m	111	30m	111
30 Month										
1	21m	70	21m	70	21m	70	21m	70	21m	70
2	21m	70	21m	70	24m	80	24m	80	24m	80
3	24m	80	24m	80	24m	80	24m	80	24m	80
4	24m	80	24m	80	30m	100	30m	100	30m	100
5	30m	100	30m	100	30m	100	30m	100	30m	100
6	30m	100	30m	100	30m	100	30m	100	30m	100

(continued)

Table 1. *(continued)*

Questionnaire items	Communication		Gross motor		Fine motor		Problem solving		Personal-social	
	Age	DQ	Age	DQ	Age	DQ	Age	DQ	Age	DQ
33 Month										
1	24m	73	21m	64	24m	73	24m	73	24m	73
2	24m	73	24m	73	30m	91	24m	73	24m	73
3	30m	91	24m	73	30m	91	24m	73	30m	91
4	30m	91	30m	91	30m	91	30m	91	30m	91
5	36m	109	30m	91	30m	91	30m	91	30m	91
6	36m	109	36m	109	30m	91	30m	91	36m	109
36 Month										
1	24m	67	24m	67	24m	67	24m	67	24m	67
2	24m	67	24m	67	24m	67	24m	67	24m	67
3	30m	83	30m	83	30m	83	30m	83	30m	83
4	30m	83	30m	83	30m	83	30m	83	30m	83
5	36m	100	36m	100	36m	100	36m	100	36m	100
6	36m	100	36m	100	36m	100	36m	100	36m	100
42 Month										
1	30m	71	30m	71	30m	71	30m	71	30m	71
2	30m	71	30m	71	30m	71	30m	71	30m	71
3	36m	86	36m	86	36m	86	36m	86	36m	86
4	36m	86	36m	86	36m	86	36m	86	36m	86
5	36–48m	86–114	36–57m	86–135	36–48m	86–114	36–57m	86–135	36–48m	86–114
6	36–49m	86–117	45–60m	107–117	42m	100	42m	100	31–49m	74–117

48 Month										
1	40–72m	88–150	36–57m	75–119	36–48m	75–100	36–48m	75–100	36–48m	75–100
2	54–60m	113–125	45–60m	94–125	36–57m	75–108	36–57m	75–119	43–60m	100–125
3	30–60m	63–125	36–48m	75–100	48–60m	100–125	36–53m	75–111	36–54m	75–113
4	48–60m	100–125	35m	73	48m	100	41–53m	85–111	48m	100
5	36–48m	75–100	36–48m	75–100	48m	100	42m	88	42–60m	88–125
6	36–49m	75–102	36–72m	75–150	48m	100	36–44m	75–92	31–49m	65–102
54 Month										
1	36–60m	66–111	35m	65	48–60m	88–111	41–53m	76–98	36–54m	66–100
2	48–60m	88–111	36–48m	66–88	48m	88	42m	77	48m	88
3	36–49m	66–91	36–48m	66–88	48m	88	36–44m	81–82	42–60m	77–111
4	36–48m	66–88	36–57m	66–106	45m	83	36–57m	82–106	36–48m	66–88
5	48m	88	36–72m	66–133	54m	100	54m	100	48–60m	88–111
6	48–59m	88–109	54–60m	100–111	48–57m	88–106	53–60m	98–111	51–66m	94–122
60 Month										
1	36–48m	60–80	36–48m	60–80	45m	75	36–57m	60–75	36–48m	60–80
2	48m	80	36–57m	60–95	54m	90	41–53m	68–88	36–54m	60–90
3	48–59m	80–98	36–72m	60–120	48–57m	80–95	54m	90	48–60m	80–100
4	54–60m	90–100	54–60m	90–100	48–60m	80–100	60m	100	51–66m	85–110
5	54–60m	90–100	60m	100	48–60m	80–100	53–60m	88–100	51–66m	85–110
6	54–60m	90–100	60–66m	100–110	54–66m	90–110	60m	100	48–62m	80–103

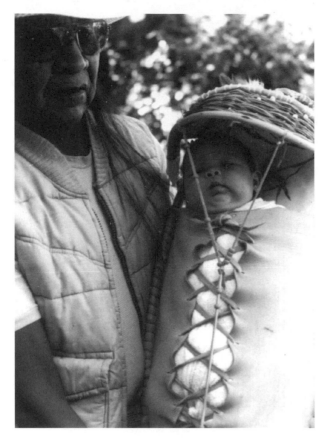

Revisions of the *Ages & Stages Questionnaires*

First Revision In response to validity and utility data gathered on the questionnaires (e.g., Brinker, Franzier, Lancelot, & Norman, 1989), the questionnaires were revised in 1991. Five types of changes were made. First, a number of items were reworded to clarify meaning. These modifications were made based on feedback from project staff, interventionists, parents, nurses, and pediatricians using the questionnaires in clinic and research environments. In most cases, the modifications entailed minimal word changes. For example, "reach for a toy" was changed to "try to get a toy"; "couch or adult chair" was changed to "furniture"; "being able to stop" was changed to "stopping"; and "stack" was changed to "stack on top of." In a few cases, examples were added or modified. For example, "Does your baby play ball with you by either rolling or throwing the ball to you?" was changed to "Does your baby either roll or throw a ball back to you so that you can return it to him?" For some items, examples were expanded to include the use of familiar and more available household objects to facilitate completion of the questionnaires by parents from diverse households. For example, "toy" and "four objects like blocks or cars" were substituted for "block" in several instances. In other cases, illustrations were added or modified to clarify the intent of the item. For example, one illustration was modified so that it was clear that the infant was using her hands for assistance rather than sitting unassisted with a straight back.

Second, modifications of a more extensive nature were made. In some cases, an item that was difficult to interpret was eliminated and replaced with another item. In all cases, the substituted items appeared on an ASQ at the previous or next interval. For example, on the 20 month questionnaire, an item in the fine motor area was eliminated and replaced with an item from the fine motor area of the 24 month questionnaire. The number and type of modifications for each questionnaire can be found in Table 2.

The third change made to revise the questionnaires was the elimination of items with a developmental quotient of 125–150. On the initial version of the questionnaires, each behavior area included one item with a developmental range of 125–150. These additional five items per questionnaire were added to provide information on parents' reported tendency to overestimate their children's developmental status (cf. Gradel, Thompson, & Sheehan, 1981; Hunt & Paraskevopoulos, 1980).

To examine how parents scored the 30 validity check items, the percentage of parents who scored these items *yes* was calculated. Table 3 indicates by

Table 2. Number of items per questionnaire with minor and major revisions

Questionnaire interval[a]	Minor wording revisions	Major revisions or substitutions
4	20	1
8	28	1
12	28	0
16	26	1
20	25	3
24	26	2
30	23	1
36	23	0

[a]The questionnaires targeting 48 and 60 months were not developed when this analysis was completed.

area the percentage of parents who selected *yes* for these items. The percentage of *yes* responses to these 30 items ranged from a low of 4% to a high of 81% (with a mean of 21%). This analysis does not support the notion that parents overestimate their children's developmental achievements. Rather, the analysis suggests that there is wide variation in the developmental achievements of children. Further support for the accuracy of parental judgments of children's developmental skills is found in an earlier study of the questionnaires (Bricker & Squires, 1989) in which interrater agreement on the questionnaires for 112 parents and several trained examiners exceeded 90%. Finally, on a number of occasions, trained examiners corroborated parental reports by observing infants and children exhibiting behaviors far above their general developmental level. For these reasons, items exceeding a DQ of 125 were eliminated from the revised questionnaires.

A fourth change was the ordering of items within each area according to their developmental order. As mentioned previously, items appeared in random developmental order within each area on the original version of the questionnaires. The five items in each area (e.g., communication, fine motor) were rearranged, beginning with the lowest age item and moving to the highest age item.

A fifth modification was the addition of the 6, 18, and 48 month questionnaires. The 6 and 18 month questionnaires were constructed by taking developmentally appropriate items from the adjacent questionnaires and adding items when necessary. The 48 month questionnaire was developed by examining a variety of tests and other developmental resources and constructing test items. The same criteria for the development of the previous questionnaires were applied to items for the 48 month questionnaire.

Table 3. The percentage of parents scoring *yes* on the 30 items with developmental quotients over 125 by area and questionnaire interval

		Percent of *yes* responses				
Questionnaire (by month)	*n*	Communication	Gross motor	Fine motor	Problem solving	Personal-social
4	625	81	27	35	24	24
8	594	14	17	40	7	12
12	562	8	40	10	7	35
16	547	15	13	10	18	10
20	472	4	39	24	25	7
24	503	13	14	44	13	14

Second Revision A second revision of the questionnaires was completed in June of 1994. Revisions were minor, and little adjustment of the items was undertaken. This revision included three types of modifications: name changes, minor modification of items, and format changes.

First, a new name, *Ages & Stages Questionnaires,*[3] was adopted to be more appealing to parents and professionals. Second, minor wording modifications were made to increase the clarity of items. For example, qualifying words such as "generally" or "usually" were eliminated. Finally, the questionnaire format was modified to be more user friendly.

Additional Intervals From 1997 to 1998, additional intervals were completed at 10, 14, 22, 27, 33, 42, 54, and 60 months. These intervals were added to make the ASQ series more comprehensive and to avoid screening children whose ages fall outside the validity "window." Validity and reliability studies were begun on the 60 month (5 year) ASQ. The remaining additional intervals (including 6 and 8 months) have not been studied; cutoff points were determined by estimating developmental quotients using age equivalencies. All items appear on questionnaires that have been empirically studied, however.

Ages & Stages Questionnaires: Social-Emotional Also in 1997, with the passage of the amendments to the Individuals with Disabilities Education Act (IDEA), came a call for early detection of social or emotional problems in young children. The *Ages & Stages Questionnaires: Social-Emotional* is a screening tool, meant to be used in conjunction with the ASQ, to identify the need for further social and emotional behavior assessment in children from 3 to 60 months of age. Eight questionnaires are available, in either English or Spanish, that address seven behavioral areas: self-regulation, compliance, communication, adaptive functioning, autonomy, affect, and interaction with people. An accompanying *User's Guide* is also available to assist professionals in the effective use of the ASQ:SE questionnaires.

DEMOGRAPHIC CHARACTERISTICS OF SAMPLES

The data reported in this section include those from questionnaires completed by parents of children between 4 and 36 months old, primarily for the Infant/Child Monitoring Project in Oregon. Additional programs, such as the Easter Seals' Watch-Me-Grow Program originating in Youngstown, Ohio, and the University of Hawaii Department of Pediatrics, have supplied data from their projects on various parameters of the questionnaires. Although gender of child data were collected in all cases, other demographic variables such as ethnicity, family income, and education level of parents were not always collected because of concerns about family privacy. We have included in our analyses children with missing demographic information.

The total number of children in the original sample was 2,008.[4] Of these, 53% (n = 1,068) were male, and 47% (n = 940) were female. Ethnicity of the sample is displayed in Table 4. Level of income of participating families is contained in Table 5. Occupational status of mother and father are contained in Tables 6 and 7, respectively. Level of education of mother and father can be

[3]The questionnaires were originally known as the Infant/Child Monitoring Questionnaires.

[4]Not all children or parents are included in all studies of the questionnaires. Most validity and reliability studies included only a subsample of children and parents. An additional 320 families participated in studies of the 48 and 60 month questionnaires.

Table 4. Ethnicity of sample

Ethnicity	*n*	Percent
Caucasian	835	64.9
African American	174	13.5
Asian/Pacific Islander	5	0.4
Native American/Alaskan	188	14.6
Latino/Hispanic	52	4.0
Biracial	33	2.6
Total	1,287	100.00

Table 5. Family income level

Income (in dollars)	*n*	Percent
Less than 5,000	125	12.70
5,001–10,000	131	13.30
10,001–15,000	120	12.20
15,001–20,000	148	15.10
20,001–25,000	141	14.30
More than 25,000	296	30.10
More than 40,000	23	2.30
Total	984	100.00

Table 6. Occupational status of mother

Mother's occupation	*n*	Percent
Student	45	4.70
Unskilled laborer	495	51.90
Semiskilled laborer	33	3.50
Skilled laborer	17	1.80
Clerical	187	19.60
Administrator	77	8.10
Manager	90	9.40
Executive	9	0.90
Total	953	100.00

Table 7. Occupational status of father

Father's occupation	*n*	Percent
Student	26	3.20
Unskilled laborer	80	10.00
Semiskilled laborer	159	19.90
Skilled laborer	113	14.10
Clerical	156	19.50
Administrator	160	20.00
Manager	75	9.40
Executive	32	4.00
Total	801	100.00

Table 8. Level of mother's education

Education level	*n*	Percent
Less than seventh grade	29	1.60
Junior high	87	4.90
Partial high school	313	17.80
High school graduate	510	29.00
Partial college	469	26.60
College graduate	233	13.20
Professional	119	6.80
Total	1,760	100.00

found in Tables 8 and 9, respectively. In some cases, when no additional clarification was given on the demographic form, it was assumed that information collected on the "primary caregiver" was the mother and on the "secondary caregiver," the father.

Between 1980 and 1988, infants with medical risk factors discharged from the neonatal intensive care unit (NICU) of a regional medical facility constituted the primary research sample included in studies by the Center on Human Development. Beginning in 1988, two additional groups of children were studied: 1) those from so-called families at environmental risk as a result of economic or social conditions; and 2) young children from nonrisk, or normative, households.

Medical Risk Sample

Subjects from the medical risk sample were infants who remained at least 3 days in a Level IV NICU needing medical care for a specific problem (e.g., respiratory distress, prematurity, low birth weight).

Environmental Risk Sample

Subjects from the environmental risk sample were infants and young children from families who met one or more of the following criteria: 1) extreme poverty (according to family income level, as defined by federal guidelines, 100% poverty level); 2) maternal age of 19 years or younger at the time of the infant's birth; 3) maternal education less than twelfth grade; and/or 4) parents who had experienced involvement with children's protective services for abuse and/or neglect of their children. Infants with medical risk factors were excluded from this sample.

Table 9. Level of father's education

Education level	*n*	Percent
Less than seventh grade	8	1.00
Junior high	10	1.20
Partial high school	70	8.40
High school graduate	239	28.60
Partial college	244	29.20
College graduate	173	20.70
Professional	91	10.90
Total	835	100.00

Table 10. Children by risk status

	Male		Female	
	n	Percent	*n*	Percent
Risk	869	81.37	751	79.89
Nonrisk	199	18.63	189	20.11
Total	1,068	100.00	940	100.00

Table 11. Ethnicity by risk status

	Nonrisk		Risk	
Ethnicity	*n*	Percent	*n*	Percent
Caucasian	108	89.30	727	62.40
African American	3	2.50	171	14.70
Asian/Pacific Islander	1	.80	4	0.30
Native American/Alaskan	4	3.30	184	15.80
Latino/Hispanic	5	4.10	47	4.00
Biracial	0	0.00	33	2.80
Total	121	100.00	1,166	100.00

Table 12. Family income by risk status

	Nonrisk		Risk	
Income (in dollars)	*n*	Percent	*n*	Percent
Less than 5,000	12	3.10	113	18.80
5,001–10,000	15	3.90	116	19.30
10,001–15,000	25	6.50	95	15.90
15,001–20,000	55	14.30	93	15.50
20,001–25,000	74	19.30	67	11.20
More than 25,000	189	47.70	113	18.80
More than 40,000	20	5.20	3	0.50
Total	384	100.00	600	100.00

Normative Sample

Subjects from the normative sample were infants and young children who met the following criteria: 1) no previous history of developmental or serious health problems as reported by parents, 2) birth at full term (greater than 37 weeks'), and 3) no assignment to a NICU.

Children are categorized by risk status in Table 10. Because of the overlap among risk factors, the two risk categories—medical and environmental—were combined into one risk category for analyses. Ethnicity by sample, income level by sample, and education level by sample are contained in Tables 11, 12, and 13. The total numbers of questionnaires completed at each age interval are listed in Table 14. The total numbers of questionnaires completed for each subject are shown in Table 15. The maximum number of questionnaires that could be completed for each subject was eight (i.e., at 4, 8, 12, 16, 20, 24, 30, and 36 months); however, for most subjects (n = 950) only one questionnaire was completed. For 198 subjects, six consecutive questionnaires were completed between 4 and 24 months. For 62, or 2% of subjects, all eight questionnaires between 4 and 36 months were completed.

Table 13. Parents' educational level

	Mother				Father			
	Nonrisk		Risk		Nonrisk		Risk	
Level	*n*	Percent	*n*	Percent	*n*	Percent	*n*	Percent
Less than seventh grade	0	0.00	29	2.10	0	0.00	8	1.70
Junior high	0	0.00	87	6.30	1	0.30	9	2.00
Partial high school	8	2.10	305	22.20	8	2.10	62	13.50
High school graduate	83	21.40	427	31.20	99	26.40	140	30.50
Partial college	127	32.80	342	24.90	100	26.70	144	31.30
College graduate	111	28.70	122	8.90	97	25.90	76	16.50
Professional	58	15.00	61	4.40	70	18.70	21	4.50
Total	387	100.00	1,373	100.00	375	100.00	460	100.00

Table 14. Total questionnaires by age interval

Age interval (in months)	*n*
4	1,500
8	1,405
12	1,185
16	1,057
20	930
24	898
30	609
36	535

Table 15. Number of questionnaires completed on each subject

Number of questionnaires	*n*	Percent
1	950	33
2	587	21
3	438	15
4	345	12
5	175	6
6	198	7
7	106	4
8	62	2
Total	2,861	100

Note: Questionnaires for which there was no demographic information are included in this analysis.

RELIABILITY

Reliability studies on the ASQ system are described here. Internal consistency analyses, including correlational analyses and Cronbach's coefficient alpha (Cronbach, 1951), are included. Test–retest reliability, interobserver reliability, and standard error of measurement are discussed.

Internal Consistency

The internal consistency of the questionnaires was addressed by examining the relationship between developmental area and overall scores. Cor-

Table 16. Correlations between area and overall score on the 10 questionnaires

Age interval (in months)	*n*	Communication	Gross motor	Fine motor	Problem solving	Personal-social
4	869	.71	.70	.81	.81	.79
8	768	.72	.76	.79	.79	.79
12	617	.75	.70	.77	.78	.83
16	502	.75	.54	.76	.75	.73
20	443	.75	.70	.66	.77	.71
24	393	.69	.63	.74	.76	.76
30	305	.76	.69	.73	.83	.69
36	248	.77	.77	.78	.83	.73
48	336	.73	.69	.82	.66	.75
60	125	.44	.58	.55	.55	.48

Note: All correlations are significant at $p < .0001$.

relational analyses and Cronbach's coefficient alpha (Cronbach, 1951) were calculated.

Pearson product moment correlation coefficients were calculated for each area score with an overall score for individual questionnaires as shown in Table 16. The overall score was obtained by adding the five developmental area scores. Correlations ranged from .70 to .81 for the 4 month ASQ, from .72 to .79 for the 8 month, from .70 to .83 for the 12 month, from .54 to .76 for the 16 month, from .66 to .77 for the 20 month, from .63 to .76 for the 24 month, from .69 to .83 for the 30 month, from .73 to .83 for the 36 month, from .66 to .82 for the 48 month, and from .44 to .58 for the 60 month. All correlations were significant at $p < .0001$.

Pearson product moment coefficient correlations between developmental area and overall scores across questionnaires are contained in Table 17. Again, all correlations were significant at $p < .0001$.

Cronbach's coefficient alpha was calculated for area scores on individual questionnaires. For the communication area, alphas ranged from .63 at 4 months to .75 at 24 months. For the gross motor area, alphas ranged from .53 at 4 months to .87 at 12 and 16 months. The fine motor area had a coefficient alpha range of .49 at 20 months to .79 at 8 months. For the problem solving area, alphas ranged from .52 at 20 months to .75 at 8 months. Finally, for the personal-social area, alphas ranged from .52 at 16 months to .68 at 12 months. Table 18 contains the standardized alphas by area and age interval.

These ranges of alphas are the result of several factors. First, the varying developmental quotients of the items that compose each area are unlikely to result in a high alpha. As a result, a child performing below criterion in a particular area will not have a static score across items within that area. Second,

Table 17. Correlations between area scores collapsing across questionnaires

Area	Communication	Gross motor	Fine motor	Problem solving	Personal-social
Communication					
Gross motor	0.46				
Fine motor	0.46	0.49			
Problem solving	0.64	0.52	0.51		
Personal-social	0.48	0.51	0.39	0.59	
Overall	0.77	0.77	0.78	0.83	0.73

N = 4,145.

Note: All correlations are significant at $p < .0001$.

Table 18. Standardized alphas by area and age interval

Age interval (in months)	*n*	Communication	Gross motor	Fine motor	Problem solving	Personal-social
4	848	0.63	0.53	0.66	0.68	0.61
8	743	0.65	0.76	0.79	0.75	0.66
12	591	0.65	0.87	0.68	0.69	0.68
16	490	0.68	0.87	0.65	0.57	0.52
20	416	0.72	0.76	0.49	0.52	0.53
24	367	0.75	0.80	0.58	0.57	0.58
30	285	0.74	0.78	0.70	0.61	0.56
36	231	0.69	0.76	0.72	0.66	0.55
48	336	0.79	0.84	0.86	0.85	0.86
60	125	0.79	0.75	0.76	0.77	0.77

the error variance in a measure is increased when a statistic uses individual items rather than an aggregated total for a calculation. In this case, the reported alphas use the actual items from each area, thus the possible error variance is increased. In contrast, the Pearson product moment correlation coefficients are a product of area totals when error variance is reduced simply because individual items are combined.

Test–Retest Reliability

Test–retest reliability was determined by comparing the results of two questionnaires completed by parents in a 2-week time period. To assess the test–retest reliability of the questionnaires, parents who brought their infants to the center for a standardized assessment completed a second identical questionnaire immediately before the standardized assessment was administered. The two questionnaires completed by parents were then compared for agreement. Test–retest reliability, measured as percentage agreement between classifications based on the questionnaires completed by 175 parents at 2-week intervals, was 94%. The standard error of measurement was .10.

Interobserver Reliability

Interobserver reliability was examined by comparing infants' classifications based on questionnaires completed by parents with the classifications based on questionnaires completed by examiners immediately after the standardized assessments, as described previously. Interobserver reliability, measured as percentage agreement between classifications based on the questionnaires completed by 112 parents and those completed by 2 examiners, was 94%. The standard error of measurement was .12. Seventy-four protocols were eliminated from this analysis because one or more test areas had two or more uncompleted items. This occurred because the professional examiner had little opportunity to observe children engaged in certain activities (e.g., eating, pretend play, adaptive skills). For example, on the 20 month ASQ, the item, "Does your child copy activities you do, such as wipe up a spill, vacuum, shave, or comb hair?" was difficult for examiners to observe and, therefore, was not scored. There is no reason to believe that any particular bias was operating in the elimination of infants from this analysis.

The reliability of the questionnaires has been studied by examining the internal consistency, test–retest reliability, and interobserver reliability of the questionnaires. Internal consistency analyses indicated strong relationships across items and within areas on the questionnaires. The questionnaires also achieved substantial test–retest and interobserver reliability. Parents' evaluations of their children using the questionnaires were consistent over time. In addition, professional examiners' agreement with parental evaluations of children using the questionnaires was consistently high.

VALIDITY

Studies of the validity of the ASQ system are described here. Relative operating characteristic (ROC) analyses; determination of screening cutoff points; and studies on concurrent validity including sensitivity, specificity, overreferral, underreferral, and positive predictive value are included.

Determination of Screening Cutoff Points

Sample The first question to be addressed was the determination of the sample to be used for calculating referral cutoff points.[5] Including both the risk and nonrisk samples is more representative and would likely provide more accurate cutoff points. The method used to test this question was an analytic technique called relative (or receiver) operating characteristic. The ROC, based on statistical decision theory, was developed in the context of electronic signal detection (Peterson, Birdsall, & Fox, 1954) and has been used in a variety of disciplines, including human perception and decision making (Green & Swets, 1966). The ROC provides estimates of the probabilities of decision outcomes by revealing the trading relationship between the true positive, true negative, false positive, and false negative probabilities that can be attained by shifting the decision criteria (i.e., cutoff points).

For this analysis, the ROC was employed to provide a single value measure of accuracy, which is reported as the area of a curve. This value represents the area of the entire graph that lies beneath the curve and can vary between .50 (when no discrimination exists) to 1.0 for perfect discrimination (when the curve follows the left and upper axes, such that the true positive proportion is 1.0 for all values of the false positive proportion). The application of the ROC to the ASQ system was to establish whether cutoff points based on the risk group, the nonrisk group, or a combined group were most accurate.

Curves were generated based on cutoff points derived from the means and standard deviations for the risk, nonrisk, and combined groups, and the areas of each curve were compared for each of the first eight questionnaires. Three cutoff points were used in the calculation of the area under the curve for each group at each questionnaire age interval: 1) 1 standard deviation below the mean, 2) 1½ standard deviations below the mean, and 3) 2 standard deviations below the mean. Each of the three points on the curve were then determined by plotting the true positive probability against the false positive probability for each cutoff point. For example, for the 12 month questionnaire, three separate ROC curves were generated, representing the risk, nonrisk, and combined groups. The ROC curve produced for the combined group using these cutoff points (i.e., 2, 1½, and 1 standard deviation) is shown in Figure 1.

To look at the differences across groups (risk, nonrisk, or combined) more effectively, the proportion of area reported for each group for each question-

[5]Cutoff points refer to the score on the questionnaires at or below which the infant/child is identified for further testing.

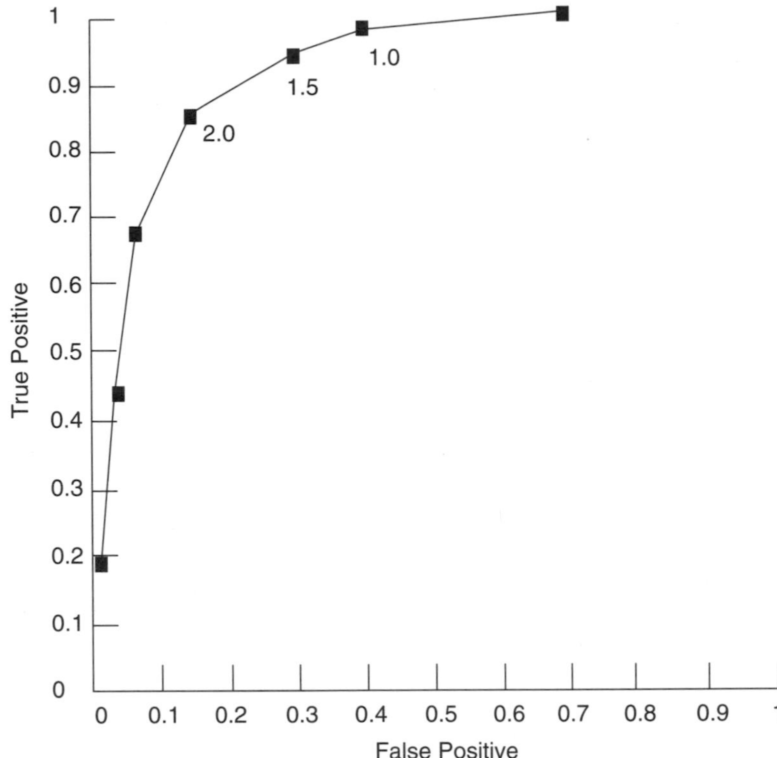

Figure 1. ROC curve generated for 12 month questionnaire combined group using 1, 1½, and 2 standard deviations.

naire was combined, and the mean area for each group was generated. The following range of areas and mean areas were found: 1) for the risk group, areas ranged from .737 to .90, with a mean of .812; 2) for the nonrisk group, areas ranged from .734 to .881, with a mean of .80; and 3) for the combined risk and nonrisk group, areas ranged from .750 to .90, with a mean of .825.

It was determined, based on the reported range of areas and mean areas by group, that points derived by using means and standard deviations from the combined risk and nonrisk group provided the most accurate cutoff points. This decision also has practical implications because agencies responsible for screening often do not know the risk status of the population to be screened. Adopting the combined risk and nonrisk referral cutoffs appeared to be most appropriate.

Cutoff Points Given that the sample used to establish cutoff points included a risk and nonrisk population, or combined group, a related question arose: Which specific cutoff point (1, 1½, or 2 standard deviations below the mean) should be used to maximize the conditional probabilities of true positive and false positive proportions? This question was addressed in two ways. First, a matrix showing the conditional probabilities that exist at each cutoff point was designed. Second, a ROC curve that graphically displayed the probabilities at each cutoff point was generated.

A matrix for each questionnaire interval was designed using the cutoff points at 2, 1½, and 1 standard deviation from the mean. This matrix included several computations that were generated using a simple contingency table.

Table 19. Cutoff points by standard deviation units and accompanying conditional probabilities for the 12 month questionnaire

Standard deviation unit(s) below the mean	Developmental area	Cutoff	Sensitivity	Specificity	True positive	False positive	Overreferral	Underreferral
2	Communication	1.54	.85	.86	.85	.13	.12	.02
	Gross motor	1.80						
	Fine motor	2.87						
	Problem solving	2.51						
	Personal-social	1.98						
1½	Communication	2.21	.95	.71	.95	.28	.25	.006
	Gross motor	2.57						
	Fine motor	3.39						
	Problem solving	3.10						
	Personal-social	2.62						
1	Communication	2.88	.97	.59	.97	.41	.36	.003
	Gross motor	3.33						
	Fine motor	3.90						
	Problem solving	3.68						
	Personal-social	3.26						

4 month ASQ

	Standardized assessment: Fail	Standardized assessment: Pass	Total
Risk	25	23	48
Developing typically	24	120	144
Total	49	143	192

Sensitivity	Specificity	False positive	True positive	False negative	Percent agreement	Under-referred	Over-referred	Percent referred	Positive predictive value
51.02%	83.92%	16.08%	51.02%	48.98%	75.52%	12.50%	11.98%	25.00%	52.08%

8 month ASQ

	Standardized assessment: Fail	Standardized assessment: Pass	Total
Risk	28	20	48
Developing typically	8	151	159
Total	36	171	207

Sensitivity	Specificity	False positive	True positive	False negative	Percent agreement	Under-referred	Over-referred	Percent referred	Positive predictive value
77.78%	88.30%	11.70%	77.78%	22.22%	86.47%	3.46%	9.66%	23.19%	58.33%

12 month ASQ

	Standardized assessment: Fail	Standardized assessment: Pass	Total
Risk	33	39	72
Developing typically	6	249	255
Total	39	288	327

Sensitivity	Specificity	False positive	True positive	False negative	Percent agreement	Under-referred	Over-referred	Percent referred	Positive predictive value
84.62%	86.46%	13.54%	84.62%	15.38%	86.24%	1.83%	11.93%	24.33%	45.83%

16 month ASQ

	Standardized assessment: Fail	Standardized assessment: Pass	Total
Risk	16	31	47
Developing typically	6	135	141
Total	22	166	188

Sensitivity	Specificity	False positive	True positive	False negative	Percent agreement	Under-referred	Over-referred	Percent referred	Positive predictive value
72.73%	81.33%	18.67%	72.73%	27.27%	80.32%	3.19%	16.49%	25.00%	34.04%

(continued)

Figure 2. Cross tabulation of agreement between combined standardized assessments and ASQ by age interval. For the 4, 8, 12, 16, and 20 month comparisons, the standardized assessment instruments used were the Bayley Scales of Infant Development (Bayley, 1969) and the Revised Gesell and Armatruda Developmental and Neurological Examination (Knobloch et al., 1980). For the 24 month comparison, these instruments and the Stanford-Binet Intelligence Scale (Thorndike et al., 1985) were used. The 30 month comparison used all of the above-mentioned instruments and the McCarthy Scales of Children's Abilities (McCarthy, 1972). The 36 month comparison used only the Gesell, the Stanford-Binet Intelligence Scale, and the McCarthy Scales of Children's Abilities. The 48 month comparison used only the McCarthy Scales of Children's Abilities. The Battelle Developmental Inventory (Newborg, Stock, Wnek, Guidubaldi, & Svinicki, 1984) was used at 60 months.

Figure 2. *(continued)*

20 month ASQ

	Standardized assessment: *Fail*	Standardized assessment: *Pass*	Total
Risk	17	13	30
Developing typically	9	119	128
Total	26	132	158

Sensitivity	Specificity	False positive	True positive	False negative	Percent agreement	Under-referred	Over-referred	Percent referred	Positive predictive value
65.38%	90.15%	9.58%	65.38%	34.62%	86.70%	5.70%	8.23%	18.99%	56.67%

24 month ASQ

	Standardized assessment: *Fail*	Standardized assessment: *Pass*	Total
Risk	12	37	49
Developing typically	3	174	177
Total	15	211	226

Sensitivity	Specificity	False positive	True positive	False negative	Percent agreement	Under-referred	Over-referred	Percent referred	Positive predictive value
80.00%	82.46%	17.54%	80.00%	20.00%	82.30%	1.33%	16.37%	21.68%	24.49%

30 month ASQ

	Standardized assessment: *Fail*	Standardized assessment: *Pass*	Total
Risk	9	19	28
Developing typically	3	113	116
Total	12	132	144

Sensitivity	Specificity	False positive	True positive	False negative	Percent agreement	Under-referred	Over-referred	Percent referred	Positive predictive value
75.00%	85.61%	14.39%	75.00%	25.00%	84.72%	2.08%	13.19%	19.44%	32.14%

36 month ASQ

	Standardized assessment: *Fail*	Standardized assessment: *Pass*	Total
Risk	9	5	14
Developing typically	1	53	54
Total	10	58	68

Sensitivity	Specificity	False positive	True positive	False negative	Percent agreement	Under-referred	Over-referred	Percent referred	Positive predictive value
90.00%	91.53%	8.47%	90.00%	10.00%	91.30%	1.45%	7.25%	20.29%	64.29%

(continued)

Figure 2. *(continued)*

48 month ASQ

	Standardized assessment		
	Fail	*Pass*	Total
Risk	7	14	21
Developing typically	2	80	82
Total	9	94	103

Sensitivity	Specificity	False positive	True positive	False negative	Percent agreement	Under-referred	Over-referred	Percent referred	Positive predictive value
77.78%	85.11%	14.89%	77.78%	22.22%	84.67%	1.94%	13.59%	20.38%	33.33%

60 month ASQ

	Standardized assessment		
	Fail	*Pass*	Total
Risk	5	0	5
Developing typically	1	24	25
Total	6	24	30

Sensitivity	Specificity	False positive	True positive	False negative	Percent agreement	Under-referred	Over-referred	Percent referred	Positive predictive value
83.33%	100.00%	0.00%	83.33%	16.67%	96.67%	3.33%	0.00%	16.67%	100.00%

Cutoff points for developmental areas were included, along with conditional probabilities that were computed based on a contingency table. A sample matrix for the 12 month questionnaire can be found in Table 19 with the following conditional probabilities: 1) sensitivity, 2) specificity, 3) true positive proportion, 4) false positive proportion, 5) overreferral, and 6) underreferral. (For definitions and computational formulas, see Chapter 6.) Cross tabulations of agreement between combined standardized assessments and the *Ages & Stages Questionnaires* by age interval can be found in Figure 2. As expected, when the cutoff becomes less conservative (i.e., 1½ or 1 standard deviation from the mean), the overreferral rate increases as the underreferral rate decreases.

Further demonstration of the trading relationship of true positive and false positive proportions as the cutoff point is adjusted is provided with the graphic representation of the ROC curve in Figure 1. It can be seen from Table 19 how the cutoff points differ in their placement on the curve. The 2 standard deviations cutoff point, although not perfect, appeared the most balanced cutoff point in terms of the true positive and false positive proportions.

For every questionnaire interval, the process of evaluation described previously was undertaken, and conditional probabilities across questionnaires were computed to arrive at a mean figure for each. These probabilities are reported in Table 20. The same trend, as described for the 12 month questionnaire, is evident in Table 20 for other questionnaire age intervals. Specifically, the sensitivity, or true positive proportion, could be maximized as the cutoff point was raised but at the expense of specificity, false positive proportions, overreferral, and underreferral.

Table 20. Mean conditional probabilities across questionnaire age intervals by cutoff point

Cutoff point (in standard deviations below the mean)	Sensitivity	Specificity	True positive	False positive	Over-referral	Under-referral
2	.75	.86	.75	.14	.12	.04
1½	.82	.74	.82	.26	.23	.03
1	.91	.60	.91	.40	.35	.01

Based on the analyses conducted using the contingency table conditional probabilities and the ROC curve, a referral cutoff point of 2 standard deviations below the mean across questionnaire intervals was recommended.[6] Because of the serial nature of the questionnaires, a child with delayed development should be identified at a test interval, even if the child is underreferred at one or two test intervals. Inherent errors will always exist when using screening tools because of the lack of an infallible criterion for measuring effectiveness, the uneven nature of early human development, and the balancing of the conditional probabilities used to determine the test's accuracy.

Concurrent Validity Concurrent validity was measured by comparing the classifications of the child's performance based on the parent-completed questionnaire with the classification of the child's performance on a professionally administered standardized test given within 29 days. The Revised Gesell and Amatruda Developmental and Neurological Examination (Knobloch et al., 1980) and the Bayley Scales of Infant Development (Bayley, 1969) were used for infants up to 30 months of age; the Stanford-Binet Intelligence Scale (Thorndike, Hagen, & Sattler, 1985) and the McCarthy Scales of Children's Abilities (McCarthy, 1972) were used for children 3–4 years old. The Battelle Developmental Inventory (BDI) (Newborg et al., 1984) was used at 60 months (5 years) of age. The child's performance on the standardized test was designated as "identified" if the child's scaled score was equal to or less than 1½ standard deviations below the mean on any scale or subscale. This scaled score (76 on the Bayley Scales of Infant Development, the McCarthy Scales of Children's Abilities, the Stanford-Binet Intelligence Scale, and the BDI; and 75 on the Gesell) was chosen because it was believed that a child scoring at or below this point was suspect for developmental delay and should be seen for further diagnostic assessment. In addition, a 1½–standard deviation delay on a standardized test meets eligibility criteria established by many states for entrance into early intervention programs (Brown & Brown, 1993).

To examine agreement between the questionnaire and the standardized measure, the child's classifications on a developmental test and a questionnaire were compared. A child was considered "identified" when his or her score fell below the cutoff point set at 2 standard deviations below the mean. One of the following four outcomes was possible:

1. Both tests classified the child as developing typically or not "identified."
2. Both tests classified the child as "identified."
3. The standardized measure indicated the child as developing typically, and the questionnaire as "identified."

[6]Agencies with sufficient resources to assess additional children can raise the cutoff points to 1½ or 1 standard deviation.

Ages & Stages Questionnaires

	Standardized assessment		
	Fail	*Pass*	Total
Risk	161	201	362
Developing typically	63	1219	1282
Total	224	1420	1644

Sensitivity	Specificity	False positive	True positive	False negative	Percent agreement	Under-referred	Over-referred	Percent referred	Positive predictive value
71.88%	85.84%	14.15%	71.88%	28.12%	83.94%	3.83%	12.22%	22.02%	44.47%

Figure 3. Cross tabulation of agreement between standardized assessments and the ASQ system across age intervals 4–48 months. The standardized assessment instruments used were the Bayley Scales of Infant Development (Bayley, 1969), the Gesell (Knobloch et al., 1980), the Stanford-Binet Intelligence Scale (Thorndike et al., 1985), and the McCarthy Scales of Children's Abilities (McCarthy, 1972).

4. The questionnaire classified the child as developing typically, and the standardized measure as "identified."

Agreement between standardized assessments and the ASQ system across questionnaires is contained in Figure 3. Contingency tables containing agreement between combined standardized assessments and the ASQ system by age interval can be found in Figure 2. Contingency tables containing agreement between individual standardized tests and the ASQ system by age interval can be found in Figure 4.

Validity with Children with Disabilities A study of the current validity of the questionnaires with a subsample of children with disabilities was undertaken. Children in this study ranged from 4 to 36 months old and were enrolled in state-funded early intervention programs for children with mild to severe disabilities. These children had received a multidisciplinary assessment and were found by professional evaluators to meet state eligibility guidelines for receiving publicly supported early intervention services. Of the 46 children whose parents completed questionnaires, 44, or 96%, were identified as in need of further assessment by the questionnaires (i.e., scored below the established cutoff points).

General Validity The validity of the ASQ system has been evaluated extensively. The concurrent validity of the questionnaires as reported in percent agreement between questionnaires and standardized assessments ranged from 76% for the 4 month ASQ to 91% for the 36 month ASQ, with 84% overall agreement. Sensitivity ranged from 51% for the 4 month ASQ to 90% for the 36 month ASQ, with 72% overall agreement. Specificity of the questionnaires ranged from 81% for the 16 month ASQ to 92% for the 36 month ASQ, with 86% overall agreement. Specificity, or the ability of the ASQ system to correctly identify typically developing children, remained high across questionnaire intervals and standardized assessments. Sensitivity, or the ability to detect delayed development, was lower, averaging 72%. In a separate analysis, however, the ability of the questionnaires to identify children with established developmental delays was high (96%).

RISK AND NONRISK GROUP COMPARISONS

Although it was determined that the combined risk and nonrisk groups provided the best sample for determining referral cutoff points, an analysis of dif-

4 Month ASQ

Bayley Scales of Infant Development

		Fail	*Pass*	
4 month ASQ	*Risk*	0	2	2
	Developing typically	0	16	16
Total		0	18	18

Revised Gesell Developmental Examination

		Fail	*Pass*	
4 month ASQ	*Risk*	25	21	46
	Developing typically	24	104	128
Total		49	125	174

Assessment	Sensitivity	Specificity	False positive rate	True positive rate	False negative rate	Percent agreement	Under-referred	Over-referred	Percent referred	Positive predictive value
BAYLEY	—	88.89%	11.11%	—	—	88.89%	0.00%	11.11%	11.11%	0.00%
GESELL	51.02%	83.20%	16.80%	51.02%	48.98%	74.14%	13.79%	12.07%	26.44%	54.35%

8 Month ASQ

Bayley Scales of Infant Development

		Fail	*Pass*	
8 month ASQ	*Risk*	3	5	8
	Developing typically	2	27	29
Total		5	32	37

Revised Gesell Developmental Examination

		Fail	*Pass*	
8 month ASQ	*Risk*	25	15	40
	Developing typically	6	124	130
Total		31	139	170

Assessment	Sensitivity	Specificity	False positive rate	True positive rate	False negative rate	Percent agreement	Under-referred	Over-referred	Percent referred	Positive predictive value
BAYLEY	60.00%	84.38%	15.63%	60.00%	40.00%	81.08%	5.41%	13.51%	21.62%	37.50%
GESELL	80.65%	89.21%	10.79%	80.65%	19.35%	87.65%	3.53%	8.82%	23.53%	62.50%

(continued)

Figure 4. Cross tabulation of agreement between the ASQ system and standardized assessment by age interval.

Figure 4. *(continued)*

12 Month ASQ

Bayley Scales of Infant Development

12 month ASQ		*Fail*	*Pass*	
	Risk	7	16	23
	Developing typically	3	139	142
Total		10	155	165

Revised Gesell Developmental Examination

12 month ASQ		*Fail*	*Pass*	
	Risk	26	23	49
	Developing typically	3	110	113
Total		29	133	162

Assessment	Sensitivity	Specificity	False positive rate	True positive rate	False negative rate	Percent agreement	Under-referred	Over-referred	Percent referred	Positive predictive value
BAYLEY	70.00%	90.00%	10.00%	70.00%	30.00%	88.48%	1.81%	9.69%	14.00%	30.43%
GESELL	89.66%	82.71%	17.29%	89.66%	10.34%	83.95%	1.85%	14.20%	30.25%	53.06%

16 Month ASQ

Bayley Scales of Infant Development

16 month ASQ		*Fail*	*Pass*	
	Risk	7	13	20
	Developing typically	1	55	56
Total		8	68	76

Revised Gesell Developmental Examination

16 month ASQ		*Fail*	*Pass*	
	Risk	9	18	27
	Developing typically	5	80	85
Total		14	98	112

Assessment	Sensitivity	Specificity	False positive rate	True positive rate	False negative rate	Percent agreement	Under-referred	Over-referred	Percent referred	Positive predictive value
BAYLEY	87.50%	80.88%	19.12%	87.50%	12.50%	81.58%	1.32%	17.11%	26.32%	35.00%
GESELL	64.29%	81.63%	18.37%	64.29%	35.71%	79.46%	4.46%	16.07%	24.11%	33.33%

20 Month ASQ

Bayley Scales of Infant Development

20 month ASQ		*Fail*	*Pass*	
	Risk	11	6	17
	Developing typically	4	51	55
Total		15	57	72

Revised Gesell Developmental Examination

20 month ASQ		*Fail*	*Pass*	
	Risk	6	7	13
	Developing typically	5	68	73
Total		11	75	86

Assessment	Sensitivity	Specificity	False positive rate	True positive rate	False negative rate	Percent agreement	Under-referred	Over-referred	Percent referred	Positive predictive value
BAYLEY	73.33%	90.38%	9.62%	73.33%	26.67%	86.57%	5.97%	7.46%	23.88%	68.75%
GESELL	54.55%	90.67%	9.33%	54.55%	45.45%	86.05%	5.81%	8.14%	15.12%	46.15%

24 Month ASQ

Bayley Scales of Infant Development

24 month ASQ		*Fail*	*Pass*	
	Risk	7	29	36
	Developing typically	1	111	112
Total		8	140	148

Revised Gesell Developmental Examination

24 month ASQ		*Fail*	*Pass*	
	Risk	5	7	12
	Developing typically	2	61	63
Total		7	68	75

Assessment	Sensitivity	Specificity	False positive rate	True positive rate	False negative rate	Percent agreement	Under-referred	Over-referred	Percent referred	Positive predictive value
BAYLEY	87.50%	79.28%	20.71%	87.50%	12.50%	79.72%	0.67%	19.59%	24.32%	19.44%
GESELL	71.43%	89.71%	10.29%	71.43%	28.57%	88.00%	2.67%	9.33%	16.00%	41.67%

(continued)

Figure 4. *(continued)*

24 Month ASQ

Stanford-Binet Intelligence Scale

		Fail	*Pass*	
24 month ASQ	*Risk*	0	1	1
	Developing typically	0	2	2
Total		0	3	3

Assessment	Sensitivity	Specificity	False positive rate	True positive rate	False negative rate	Percent agreement	Under-referred	Over-referred	Percent referred	Positive predictive value
STANFORD-BINET	—	66.67%	33.33%	—	—	66.67%	0.00%	33.33%	33.33%	0.00%

30 Month ASQ

Bayley Scales of Infant Development

		Fail	Pass	
30 month ASQ	*Risk*	7	16	23
	Developing typically	3	98	101
Total		10	114	124

Revised Gesell Developmental Examination

		Fail	Pass	
30 month ASQ	*Risk*	2	1	3
	Developing typically	0	5	5
Total		2	6	8

McCarthy Scales of Children's Abilities

		Fail	Pass	
30 month ASQ	*Risk*	0	0	0
	Developing typically	0	4	4
Total		0	4	4

Assessment	Sensitivity	Specificity	False positive rate	True positive rate	False negative rate	Percent agreement	Under-referred	Over-referred	Percent referred	Positive predictive value
BAYLEY	70.00%	85.96%	14.03%	70.00%	30.00%	84.67%	2.41%	12.90%	18.54%	30.43%
GESELL	100.00%	83.33%	16.67%	100.00%	0.00%	87.50%	0.00%	12.50%	37.50%	66.67%
McCARTHY	—	100.00%	0.00%	—	—	100.00%	0.00%	0.00%	0.00%	—

(continued)

Figure 4. *(continued)*

36 Month ASQ

McCarthy Scales of Children's Abilities

36 month ASQ		*Fail*	*Pass*	
	Risk	0	0	0
	Developing typically	0	5	5
Total		0	5	5

Revised Gesell Developmental Examination

36 month ASQ		*Fail*	*Pass*	
	Risk	9	2	11
	Developing typically	1	19	20
Total		10	21	31

Assessment	Sensitivity	Specificity	False positive rate	True positive rate	False negative rate	Percent agreement	Under-referred	Over-referred	Percent referred	Positive predictive value
McCARTHY	—	100.00%	0.00%	—	—	100.00%	0.00%	0.00%	0.00%	—
GESELL	90.00%	90.48%	9.52%	90.00%	10.00%	90.32%	3.23%	6.45%	35.48%	81.82%

36 Month ASQ

Stanford-Binet Intelligence Scale

36 month ASQ		*Fail*	*Pass*	
	Risk	0	3	3
	Developing typically	0	30	30
Total		0	33	33

Assessment	Sensitivity	Specificity	False positive rate	True positive rate	False negative rate	Percent agreement	Under-referred	Over-referred	Percent referred	Positive predictive value
STANFORD-BINET	—	90.91%	9.09%	—	—	90.91%	0.00%	9.09%	9.09%	0.00%

48 Month ASQ

McCarthy Scales of Children's Abilities

		Fail	*Pass*	
48 month ASQ	*Risk*	7	14	21
	Developing typically	2	80	82
Total		9	94	103

Assessment	Sensitivity	Specificity	False positive rate	True positive rate	False negative rate	Percent agreement	Under-referred	Over-referred	Percent referred	Positive predictive value
McCARTHY	77.78%	85.11%	14.89%	77.78%	22.22%	84.67%	1.94%	13.59%	20.38%	33.33%

60 Month ASQ

Battelle Developmental Inventory

		Fail	*Pass*	
60 month ASQ	*Risk*	5	0	5
	Developing typically	1	24	25
Total		6	24	30

Assessment	Sensitivity	Specificity	False positive rate	True positive rate	False negative rate	Percent agreement	Under-referred	Over-referred	Percent referred	Positive predictive value
BATTELLE DEVELOPMENTAL INVENTORY	83.33%	100.00%	0.00%	83.33%	16.67%	96.67%	3.33%	0.00%	16.67%	100.00%

ferences between these groups provided interesting information regarding comparative group performances. Item analyses and analyses of differences between groups by questionnaires were undertaken.

Item Analyses

Item analyses of risk and nonrisk group differences are presented in this section. The performance of the nonrisk group was believed to exceed that of the risk group on individual questionnaire items. To address this question, scoring of items in developmental areas on the eight original questionnaires (4, 8, 12, 16, 20, 24, 30, and 36 month intervals) was compared and a mean score for each was generated. A total of 240 items were examined.

Table 21 presents for each skill area the number of items in which 1) the mean score of the risk group exceeded the nonrisk group, 2) the mean score of the nonrisk group exceeded the risk group, and 3) the mean scores of the two groups were equal. The number of risk and nonrisk subjects included in this analysis was 6,377 and 1,682, respectively. From a total of 231 items, there were 19%, or only 43 items, in which mean scores for the risk group exceeded the mean scores for the nonrisk group.

Table 22 shows the same comparison by questionnaire interval. The number of items in which the risk group mean scores exceeded, were less

Table 21. Number of items by area on which the mean score for the risk group was greater than, less than, or equal to the nonrisk group

Area	Greater	Less	Equal
Communication	10	34	0
Gross motor	6	40	0
Fine motor	7	37	1
Problem solving	7	39	2
Personal-social	13	35	0
Total	43	185	3

Risk $n = 6{,}377$.
Nonrisk $n = 1{,}682$.
Note: Nine items in these developmental areas were changed between revisions and, therefore, were not included.

Table 22. Number of items by questionnaire in which the mean score for the risk group was greater than, less than, or equal to the nonrisk group

Age interval (in months)	*n*	Greater	Less	Equal
4	1,501	12	18	0
8	1,405	4	24	1
12	1,185	6	24	0
16	1,057	6	23	0
20	930	3	24	0
24	898	8	19	1
30	566	3	24	1
36	517	1	29	0
Total	8,059	43	185	3

Risk $n = 6{,}377$.
Nonrisk $n = 1{,}682$.
Note: Nine items in these developmental areas were changed between revisions and, therefore, were not included.

than, or equal to the nonrisk group are displayed for each questionnaire age interval. As can be seen in Table 22, the 43 items on which the risk group's mean score exceeded the nonrisk group are distributed across intervals with the greatest frequency at 4 months.

Analysis of Group Differences for the Risk and Nonrisk Groups

To test for differences between the risk and nonrisk groups, the five area scores (e.g., communication, fine motor) for the questionnaire intervals (e.g., 4, 8, 12, 16, 20, and 24 months) were compared. A 2 × 6 (group × questionnaire) mixed model multivariate analysis of variance (MANOVA) was conducted. Status of the subject as either risk or nonrisk was entered as a between-subjects factor, while questionnaire interval was entered as a within-subjects variable. Any cases with incomplete data for the within-subjects variable were deleted from this analysis, leaving 249 remaining cases spanning the 4 to 24 month intervals. Because cell sizes in this design were unequal, an unweighted means or regression approach was used in the analysis of these data (Tabachnick & Fidell, 1989) using SAS GLM (SAS Institute, 1990).

With the use of Wilks's criterion, the combined dependent variables were significantly affected only by the interaction of risk status and test interval, $F(25, 4567) = 2.27$, $p < .0005$, but not by either risk status or test interval independently. The results reflected a very small association between this interaction term and the combined dependent variables ($\eta^2 = .05$). Because the focus of this analysis was the relationship between risk status and scores on the questionnaires and the main effect of risk status was not significant, follow-up analyses were not performed.

These analyses suggested that differences between groups were minimal and not consistent across questionnaire age intervals or across areas. These analyses support the decision to combine risk and nonrisk groups for determining cutoff points as well as for determining the validity and reliability of the questionnaires.

Analyses of differences between nonrisk and risk groups yielded interesting comparisons. As predicted, the nonrisk group had more items whose mean score exceeded those for the risk group. However, results of the 2 × 6 (group × questionnaire) MANOVA suggested no consistently significant differences between groups. The decision to combine risk and nonrisk groups to determine cutoff points using ROC analysis was further supported by multivariate analysis described previously.

REFERENCES

Bayley, N. (1969). *Bayley Scales of Infant Development.* San Antonio, TX: The Psychological Corporation.

Bricker, D., & Squires, J. (1989). The effectiveness of parental screening of at-risk infants: The infant monitoring questionnaires. *Topics in Early Childhood Special Education, 9*(3), 67–85.

Brinker, R., Franzier, W., Lancelot, B., & Norman, J. (1989). Identifying infants from the inner city for early intervention. *Infants and Young Children, 2*(1), 49–58.

Brown, W., & Brown, C. (1993). Defining eligibility for early intervention. In W. Brown, S.K. Thurman, & L.F. Pearl (Eds.), *Family-centered early intervention with infants and toddlers: Innovative cross-disciplinary approaches* (pp. 21–42). Baltimore: Paul H. Brookes Publishing Co.

Cohen, M., & Gross, P. (1979). *Developmental resources: Behavioral sequences for assessment and program planning* (Vols. I & II). New York: Grune & Stratton.

Cronbach, L. (1951). Coefficient alpha and the internal structure of tests. *Psychometrika, 16*(3), 297–334.

Gradel, K., Thompson, M., & Sheehan, R. (1981). Parental and professional agreement in early childhood assessment. *Topics in Early Childhood Special Education, 1,* 31–40.

Green, D., & Swets, J. (1966). *Signal detection theory and psychophysics.* New York: John Wiley & Sons.

Hunt, J., & Paraskevopoulos, J. (1980). Children's psychological development as a function of the accuracy of their mothers' knowledge of their abilities. *Journal of Genetic Psychology, 136,* 285–298.

Knobloch, H., Stevens, F., & Malone, A.F. (1980). *Manual of developmental diagnosis: The administration and interpretation of the Revised Gesell and Amatruda Developmental and Neurological Examination.* New York: Harper & Row.

McCarthy, D. (1972). *McCarthy Scales of Children's Abilities.* San Antonio, TX: The Psychological Corporation.

MECCA. (no date). *MinNesota Interactive Readability Approximation Program.* Lauderdale, MN: Author.

Newborg, J., Stock, J.R., Wnek, L., Guidubaldi, J., & Svinicki, J. (1984). *Battelle Developmental Inventory.* Chicago: Riverside.

Peterson, W., Birdsall, T., & Fox, W. (1954). Trans. IRE Prof. Group Inf. Theory PGIT-4, 171.

SAS Institute, Inc. (1990). *SAS/STAT user's guide* (Vol. 2, Vers. 6). Cary, NC: Author.

Tabachnick, R., & Fidell, L. (1989). *Using multivariate statistics* (2nd ed.). New York: Harper & Row.

Thorndike, R., Hagen, E., & Sattler, J. (1985). *Stanford-Binet Intelligence Scale* (4th ed.). Chicago: Riverside.

INDEX

Page numbers followed by "t" denote tables; those followed by "f" denote figures.